放射性セシウムが生殖系に与える医学的社会学的影響

チェルノブイリ原発事故 その人口「損失」の現実

ユーリ・I・バンダジェフスキー／N・F・ドウボバヤ [著]
久保田 護 [訳]

合同出版

本書は、放射性核種の長期的な影響下でのヒトの生殖過程を扱っている。

　体内に取り込まれたセシウム137が、妊娠と胎児の発育をつかさどる男女の生殖システムに与える影響について、動物実験を含む長期間の臨床的・病理学的観察から得たデータを提示した。チェルノブイリ原子力発電所事故で被災したウクライナの地域の人びとの出生率と生殖損失の結果を疫学的に考察した。

　本書で示されたデータは、住民の生殖健康に対する放射線のほんとうの影響を調査し、現在の人口問題を効果的に解決するのに役立つであろう。

Ⓒ Yu・I・バンダジェフスキー＋N・F・ドゥボバヤ、2011

目　次

まえがき …………………………………………………………………………… 5

第1部　体内に取り込まれたセシウム137とヒトの生殖過程 …………… 7

1.1　チェルノブイリ原発事故以前と以降の
　　　ベラルーシ共和国の放射能汚染と人口統計の状況　7
1.2　放射性セシウムが体内に取り込まれる条件での女性生殖器官の病態　12
1.3　放射性セシウムが体内に取り込まれた状況での男性生殖器官の変化　16
1.4　放射性セシウムがもたらす突然変異誘発作用　18
1.5　妊娠中および授乳期間中における放射性核種の体内取り込みの特徴　20
1.6　放射性セシウムの体内取り込みにともなう出生前と出生後の発育の病理　23
　　　1.6.1　体内に取り込まれたセシウム137量を考慮したヒトの先天性障害の評価　23
　　　1.6.2　妊娠中に放射性セシウムを体内に取り込んだ実験動物での胚胎児発生　27
1.7　胎盤の放射性セシウムの取り込み　36
1.8　放射性セシウムを取り込んだ母—胎児系の内分泌の相互関係　37
1.9　胎児と新生児の放射能毒性症候群　40

第2部　チェルノブイリ原発事故で被災した
　　　　ウクライナ住民の生殖に関する健康状態 ………………………… 51

2.1　放射能汚染郡の出生率の動向　51
2.2　人びとの生殖損失の特性評価と出生率の変遷への関与　60

むすび ……………………………………………………………………………… 65

付　録　CONSEQUENCE OF THE CHERNOBYL DISASTER:
　　　　REPRODUCTION OF HUMAN BEING IN CONDITION OF
　　　　RADIATION EXPOSURE ………………………………………… 67

[**本書について**]

＊本書の原書は以下の通りである。

　　　Ю. И. Бандажевский, Н. Ф. Дубовая, "Последствия Чернобыльской катастрофы: репродукция человека в условиях радиационного воздействия", Координационный аналитический центр «Экология и здоровье», Киев, 2011.

＊本書刊行にあたって、原著者であるバンダジェフスキー博士了承のもと、別途、合同出版編集部で英訳文を作成し、巻末付録として併載した。

＊日本語版の本文中［　］内に付記されているリファレンス番号は、巻末英訳文中の各部リファレンスに対応している。ただし、リファレンスはロシア語、およびウクライナ語、英語原文のまま。
　　第1部リファレンス：114〜120ページ
　　第2部リファレンス：134〜135ページ

装　幀　守谷義明＋六月舎
DTP　ギャラップ

まえがき

　本書は、1986年のチェルノブイリ原発事故の医学的影響を主題としている。著者らは、放射能汚染地域に住んでいる人びとの生殖の問題を明らかにしようと、ともに力を尽してきた。

　子孫を残すことは人類の主な課題のひとつであるが、チェルノブイリ原発事故の被災国では、とりわけ緊急を要する問題となっている。

　ベラルーシ、ウクライナ、ロシアの人口の動態は今や破局的である。この20年間、これらの国は人口が急速に減少している。その主な原因は、高い死亡率と低い出生率にある。この現象を、喫煙の習慣やアルコール依存症のような好ましくない社会現象、あるいは、低い生活水準に結びつけようとする試みがある。

　しかし、この試みは、地球の全生物に与えている放射線の強い影響を考慮していない。旧ソ連のヨーロッパ地域の人びとは、1960年代から放射性物質に直面し、チェルノブイリ原発事故が加わって、50年ものあいだ、放射性物質にさらされてきた。環境にもっとも広がっている放射性物質はセシウム137であり、食品を通じて人体に入り込んでいる。

　著者らは、放射線が人体に与える影響という観点から、医学界や科学界が現在の人口問題に注目することを望んでいる。

　本書の第1部では、放射性セシウムが体内に取り込まれた際の男女の生殖器官、および子宮内での胎児の発育の過程を、臨床所見、病理データ、検査データの分析、動物実験の結果を用いて明らかにする。

　第2部では、チェルノブイリ原発事故で被災したウクライナの汚染地域の住民の出生率と「生殖損失」の疫学的研究の結果を述べた。

　著者らは、読者、とくに環境要因が人体に与える影響を研究する医学者や研究者が本書のデータに注目し、放射能で汚染された住民の健康を維持する手段の開発に役立ててくださることを期待している。

第1部
体内に取り込まれたセシウム137と
ヒトの生殖過程

1.1 チェルノブイリ原発事故以前と以降の
ベラルーシ共和国の放射能汚染と人口統計の状況

いつの時代でも社会が直面するもっとも実際的な問題のひとつは、将来の世代に生命をつないでゆくことである。いいかえれば、先祖のよりよい形質を持つ子孫を産み出すことである。

ベラルーシ共和国では最近10年間、この問題の適切な解決がみつかっていない。出生率が急速に下がり、子どもの死亡率と有病率が上がり、異常や先天性奇形を持つ子どもも増えている。どうしてこうなったのかと思うのも当然だ。みんなが貧乏になって、妊娠前や妊娠中の女性の食事や医療サービスが悪くなったせいか？ それとも、おびただしい人工因子の影響だろうか？と人びとが思うのも当然だ。

ベラルーシ共和国では最近、死亡率が出生率の1.6倍になっているが、生活水準の低下が人びとの生殖過程に及ぼす影響という問題に取りくみ、歴史を振り返ったとしても、戦争や疫病といった人類がもっとも困窮したときですら、このようなことになったことはなかった。

20世紀は人類に多くの苦しみと問題をもたらした。核技術の開発は、1950年代以降、人びとの生活圏をそれまで地球になかった新しい放射性元素によってひどく汚染してしまった。

その新しい元素のひとつが、半減期30年の長寿命放射性核種セシウム137である。これは、放射性廃棄物とともに、あるいは核爆発の生成物とともに生活圏に入り込んでくる[40]。

原子炉と使用済み核燃料の再処理工場が、放射性廃棄物の発生源である。原子炉の気体廃棄物のなかで、セシウム137はおもにキセノン137から生まれ、液体廃棄物の構成部分として環境に入り込んでくる。

しかし、セシウム 137 が生活環境に最悪の汚染をもたらすのは核爆発、あるいは、1986 年のチェルノブイリのような原発事故である。

　発生した莫大な熱エネルギーの流れは、核反応生成物を成層圏まで巻き上げた。核反応生成物は、気流の作用で遠くまで運ばれ（成層圏と対流圏で）、事故が発生した場所とは無関係に、地球上のあらゆる場所に降下した。

　物理学的に厳密にいうと、セシウム 137 はベータ線を放射し、その娘核種バリウム 137 が半減期 2.55 分でガンマ線を放射する。

　ベラルーシを含む旧ソ連のヨーロッパ地域では、1963 年からセシウム 137 を記録しはじめた。人間の食料と動物の飼料中のセシウム 137 を測定した手持ちの科学資料によれば、チェルノブイリ原発事故以前において、セシウム 137 の地上への降下量がもっとも多かったのは、その 1963 年であったことがわかる[40]。

　この時期、ベラルーシの人びとの体内にセシウム 137 を高濃度で蓄積させたおもな食品は、牛乳、乳製品、パン、牛肉、豚肉である。とくに、牛肉のセシウム 137 濃度は、1967 年から 1970 年にわたってソ連保健省生物物理研究所がベラルーシのポレシエ地域で調査した結果によると、700 ～ 8300 ピコキュリー（pCi）/kg［訳注：25.9 ～ 307.1Bq/kg］で、ゴメリ州の多くの村では、住民の 1 日分の食料中に平均 2059pCi/kg［訳注：76.18Bq/kg］が検出された[40]。

　このように、チェルノブイリ事故のずっと前から（20 年以上）、ベラルーシ共和国の人びとは放射性元素、とくにセシウム 137 の影響を受けていた。

　2000 年以前には、この地域の人びとのために、食物のなかのセシウム 137 の濃度がどの程度になるかについての科学的な予測もおこなわれていた[40]。1986 年のチェルノブイリ原発 4 号炉の事故で、1 億 8000 万キュリー以上の放射性物質が大気中に放出されてしまった（原子炉のすぐ近くに放出された数トンの核燃料を除いて）。ベラルーシ、ウクライナ、ロシアとほかのヨーロッパ諸国の広大な領域が、ヨウ素 131、セシウム 137 と 134、ストロンチウム 90、プルトニウム 239 といった放射性核種によって汚染された[43]。公的な基準からみても、それらの放射性物質の食物中含有量は非常に多い。1966 年の時点で、ゴメリ州では、食物から 1 日あたり 9063.9 ～ 1 万 4280.3 ピコキュリー［訳注：335 ～ 528Bq］のセシウム 137 を摂取しても許容範囲内だと思われていた。

　放射性セシウムで汚染される前は、ベラルーシの人口状況は順調だった。第二次大戦直後の困窮した時代ですら、出生率が死亡率をかなり上まわって

いた。1960年にベラルーシの人口自然増加率は17.8パーミル（‰）となり、第二次大戦後ではもっとも高い値を記録した。ところが、1965年以降は、死亡率が高くなる一方で、出生率が年々低下していった。1985年には、人口自然増加率は5.9‰にまで低下した。1986年にチェルノブイリ原発事故が起きると、ベラルーシの人口自然増加率はさらに低下した。そして、1993年以降、死亡率がとうとう出生率を上まわるようになり、人口自然増加率はマイナス（負）の値をとるようになってしまった[41]。出生率がどんどん下がり、一方で死亡率は上がった。このため、人口自然増加率は1999年にマイナス4.9‰、2002年はマイナス5.9‰、2003年にはマイナス5.5‰、2005年にはマイナス5.9‰となった[41, 42, 50]。

　1994年から2008年にかけて、ベラルーシの人口は60万7400人も減少した。これは総人口が5.9％も減少したことを意味する。そして2009年初頭に総人口は967万1900人にまで減った。15歳以下の子どもの減少にはとくに注目すべきだ。2000年から2009年のあいだに、29万人も減ったのだ[53]。

　保健省の統計データをみると、ベラルーシの人びとの健康状態が極めて悪いことがわかる。ベラルーシ共和国の多くの州とミンスク市では、1990年から2004年までに先天性障害を持つ子どもの登録数がどんどん増えている。例外はグロドノ州とビテブスク州である（表1.1.1）。しかし、グロドノ州とビテブスク州でも1990年から2004年の間、出生率が急速に低下した。ビテブスク州では、出生率が13.8‰から7.8‰まで低下した。これらの州でも人びとの生殖が大きく低下したことがわかる。

　2000年から2008年にかけて、ベラルーシ共和国では先天性奇形や発育異常のある新生児の数が10万出生につき359.5から558.7に増加した[50-55]。

　ベラルーシ共和国の人びとの生殖に非常に重大な問題が生じていることを、先天性奇形の増加と出生率の低下が示している。このことと、死亡率の加速的な上昇によって、人口が破局的に減少していることの説明ができる。人びとは、自分たちの本当の健康状態を知らされてはいない。出生率が低下したのは、子どもをもうける動機が欠けているのであって、子どもを作る能力が失われているからではないと、人びとに説明できるものなら、先天性障害を持つ子どもの数に関する統計データに対して、反論を持ち出せないはずである。しかし本当は、生殖能力が失われているがゆえに子どもができないケースの方がはるかに多いのだ。

表 1.1.1　初めて先天性奇形を指摘された子どもの 10 万出生あたりの数

州　名	1990年	1999年	2003年	2004年
ブレスト州	59.5	128.0	115.9	86.2
ビテブスク州	48.3	50.3	—	39.9
ゴメリ州	38.9	70.6	—	86.8
グロドノ州	72.7	91.0	—	45.9
モギレフ州	52.1	80.5	—	90.7
ミンスク州	57.3	104.5	—	140.2
ミンスク市	92.2	128.8	240.5	217.1

　現在、ベラルーシでは疫学的にみて非常に多くの先天性障害児が生まれている。もはや学会で高い地位にある学者たちがふたつの陣営にわかれて論争している場合ではないのだ。先天性奇形の新生児が、ベラルーシ共和国のとくにチェルノブイリ原発事故の汚染地域で増えていることについては、明確な唯一の結論しか下すことができない。そして、ある研究所のスタッフたちも同じ結論に至り、科学的な公式報告をした[35, 36, 37]。

　しかし、原子力ロビーと旧ソ連の代議士、とくにベラルーシ共和国の議員たちにとって、この結論は都合の悪いものだった。そこで彼らは、傑出した遺伝学者であり、また奇形学の教授でもあるＧ・Ｉ・ラジューク教授が率いていた、先天性・遺伝性疾患研究所を閉鎖してしまった。この研究所は旧ソ連により創設され、ヒトの先天性疾患の病理的問題を長年にわたって科学的に広範に研究し、現状の統計的分析もおこなってきた唯一の研究機関であった。

　ベラルーシには現在、先天性疾患の発生原因に関する問題に十分な対応のできる学術組織が存在しない。数世代にわたる科学者たちによって築かれた学派は消滅してしまった。権力者たち、つまり原子力ロビーにとっては、政府には医学的知識がない方が好都合なのだ。

　このようなことは驚くに値しない。国連機関の国際原子力機関（ＩＡＥＡ）は、世界保健機関（ＷＨＯ）を長年にわたり牛耳ってきた。そして、1959 年、放射線被曝が人びとの健康に与える影響に関するデータは開示しないという協定を、ＷＨＯに押しつけた。世界中のすべての人びとの健康と生命よりも、この協定のほうが大事なのだろうか？

　公的機関に登録された先天性奇形は、この放射性物質による子宮内発育障害の氷山の一角にすぎない。子どもの体が発育し、臓器と器官系が形成され

る大事な時期に、セシウム 137 やほかの放射性物質に絶えずさらされていれば、成人後、必然的に身体の不調に悩まされると考えざるを得ない。

　突発性の心停止による成人の死亡例が多いことについて、ここで述べておくべきであろう。出生前後の発育過程で心臓の構成要素の形成が障害されることが、真の病因であるケースもある。心臓の形成障害を示唆するものとして、子どもの心筋の電気生理学的過程の異常が記録されている。子どもの心電図異常の発生頻度と体内のセシウム 137 濃度のあいだに相関があることが確認されている [45, 46, 47]。

　ただし、子どもの心電図異常をもたらす病変は、子どもが死亡する直接の病因とはならない。しかし、この異常は、ほかの病気の経過にはかなり悪影響を与えることもある。その一例としてウィルス性感染症で死亡したチェルノブイリゾーンの乳児のケースを挙げることができる。この症例は心不全を併発し、それが死因となった。ウィルスが直接的に心臓を侵したことが心筋障害の原因になったが、それ以外に放射性セシウムが心筋に入り込んで悪影響を与えていた面もあった。放射線被曝の影響で心血管系の異常と免疫系の異常が誘導され、病気になることもある。しかし、残念なことに、このことが考慮されることはまったくない。

　チェルノブイリ原発事故の汚染地域の人びとの切迫した状況、すなわち、第 1 部で取り扱うかれらの生殖障害を考慮し、1990 年～ 1999 年までゴメリ国立医大のスタッフを率いておこなった臨床研究、動物実験、放射線測定の結果を分析した。そして体内に取り込まれたセシウム 137 が生殖過程に与える影響を明らかにすることに専念した。

　以前発表した研究 [3, 5, 6, 7] と同じアプローチの仕方をとって、この問題に取り組んだ。

　　1 ）体内に取り込まれた放射性物質の計測値を考慮して医学的・生物学的な影響を評価する。
　　2 ）病理過程を臨床的に研究し、さらに動物実験でその疾患モデルを作成する（臨床と動物実験によるアプローチ）
　　3 ）個別の臓器や器官系を研究することと並行して、身体全体に起きている構造上の変化、機能的・代謝的な変化を研究する。
　　4 ）身体の統合機能の不調という視点から病変の重症度を評価する。このようなアプローチの仕方によって別々の臓器に起きている病変を互

いに関連づけて考えることができるようになる。

1.2 放射性セシウムが体内に取り込まれる条件での女性生殖器官の病態

　放射性セシウムが体内に取り込まれると子宮内では胎児の発育に異常が出る。そのことを述べる前に、このときの女性生殖器の状態について述べておく必要がある。女性生殖器官が体外からの放射線被曝によって傷つけられやすいことは、30年以上前から多くの研究によって科学的に明らかになっている[9]。しかし、現在の環境状況では、放射線による体外からの被曝の影響ではなく、体内に取り込まれた放射性物質が長時間かけて作用し、女性生殖器にどのような変化をもたらすのかということを分析する必要がある。そこで、性ホルモンの産生と体内に取り込まれた放射性セシウムの濃度を考慮しながら、生殖年齢の女性の健康状態を評価した。

　女性の体内でセシウム137濃度が40Bq/kgを超えると、月経周期のさまざまな時期で性ホルモン産生の逆転が起きることが明らかになった。そのため月経周期も当然異常になった。具体的には、第一相（卵胞期）でプロゲステロン濃度の上昇と、エストラジオール濃度の低下がみられる一方、第二相（黄体期）ではプロゲステロン濃度の低下と、エストラジオール濃度の上昇がみられた（図1.2.1、1.2.2、1.2.3、1.2.4）。

　これらの女性ホルモンの産生異常は、女性生殖器の病気の原因になるのみならず、不妊症の原因にもなる。女性ホルモンが正常に分泌されていれば、妊娠中のプロセスや母体と胎児のあいだに起きる相互作用に対応するため、子宮粘膜と女性生殖器官の準備態勢を整えることができる。しかし、女性ホルモン産生異常があれば、子宮粘膜と女性生殖器官の準備態勢を整えることができず不妊症となってしまう[34]。

　このことは、雑種の白ラットによる動物実験でも確認された。体内のセシウム137の平均濃度が53.30 ± 6.28Bq/kg（対照群は14.05 ± 3.31Bq/kg）になると、発情期の血中プロゲステロン濃度（23.96 ± 6.94nmol/l）が対照群（61.01 ± 15.66Bq/kg）よりも低くなる。そして子宮壁の厚さ（13.91 ± 0.99慣用単位）

図 1.2.1　月経周期第1相でのエストラジオール濃度

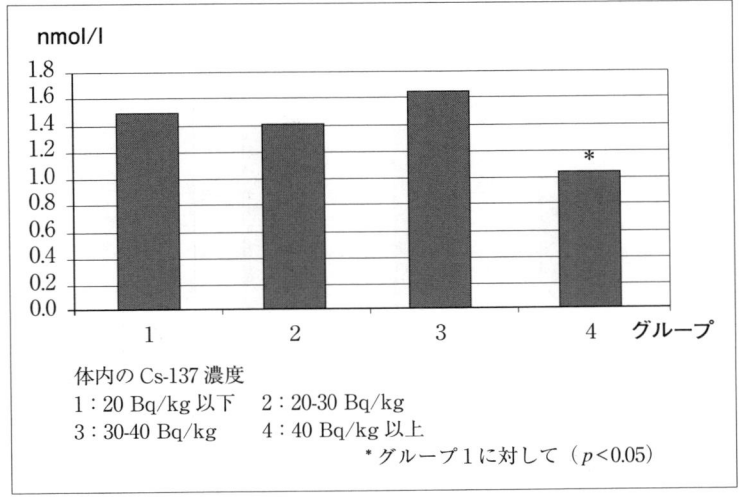

体内の Cs-137 濃度
1：20 Bq/kg 以下　2：20-30 Bq/kg
3：30-40 Bq/kg　4：40 Bq/kg 以上
＊グループ1に対して（$p<0.05$）

図 1.2.2　月経周期第1相でのプロゲステロン濃度

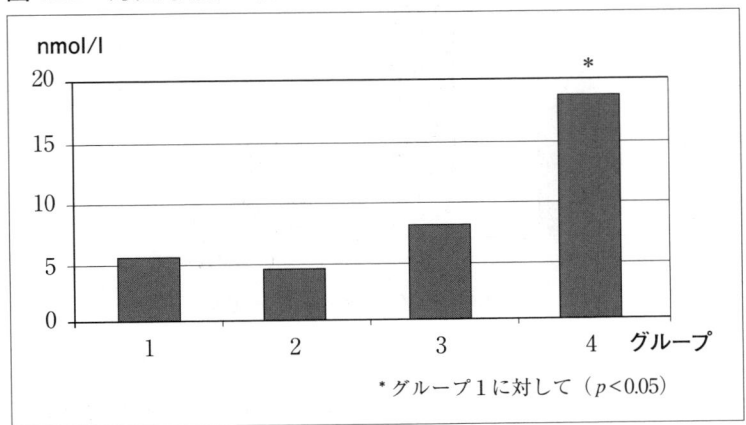

＊グループ1に対して（$p<0.05$）

は対照群（16.57 ± 0.52 慣用単位）よりも薄くなる。この実験ではラットの卵巣も調べている。しかし、第二次を含むさまざまな発育段階の卵胞数が対照群より統計的に有意に減少しているということはなかった[34]。

　しかし、ヨウ素 131 とセシウム 137 が体内に大量に取り込まれると、2つの放射性物質の影響が重なりあって卵子の形成が抑制されることが、多くの研究から明らかになっている[2]。6カ月と12カ月の長期観察では、ヨウ素

図 1.2.3　月経周期第 2 相でのエストラジオール濃度

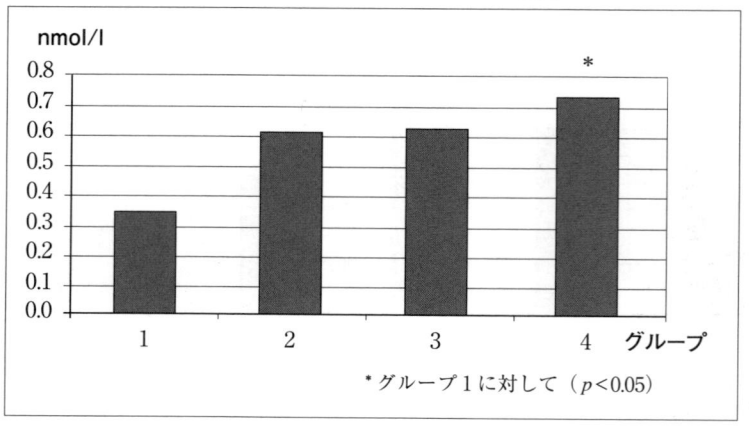

＊グループ1に対して（$p<0.05$）

図 1.2.4 月経周期第 2 相でのプロゲステロン濃度

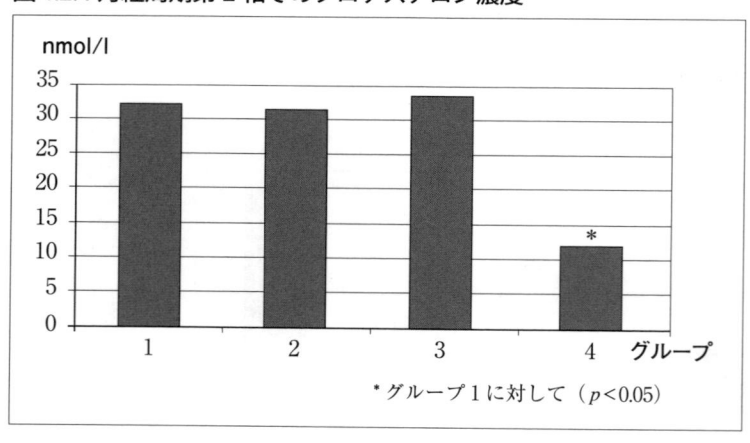

＊グループ1に対して（$p<0.05$）

131とセシウム137が体内に大量に取り込まれると、卵巣内で破壊的な病変が進行し、卵胞の総数が53％も減少することが示された。I・N・ヤゴブディクの研究によれば、体内に放射性セシウムが取り込まれると、その影響で女性の体内のホルモン産生に大きな変化が起きる[29]。そして、さまざまな神経-ホルモン分泌間の制御が障害されることが明らかになった[29]。

　若い女性の体内に放射性セシウムが取り込まれ、長いあいだその悪影響を受けると、ホルモン産生の恒常性が障害されることが明らかになった。具体的には、相対的あるいは絶対的な低プロゲステロン血症（血液中のプロゲス

テロン濃度が低下）が、高エストロゲン血症（血液中のエストロゲン濃度が上昇）と高テストステロン血症（血液中のテストステロン濃度が上昇）を背景として起きてくる。

体内のセシウム137濃度が50Bq/kg以上になると、若い女性に起きる性ホルモンの産生異常は顕著になる。体内のセシウム137濃度が50Bq/kg以上の場合、検査した女性6人にひとりに排卵がみられなかった。このように、放射性セシウムが体内に取り込まれると、その影響で月経周期の黄体期不全と無排卵症が起きる。これらはホルモン産生の制御プロセスにおける異常を反映している。

最終的な結論として、無排卵症と黄体機能不全により不妊症となる。放射性物質の汚染地域で出生率が低下している主な原因のひとつは不妊症であると私たちは考えている。

体内に取り込まれた放射性セシウムが、長い年月をかけて女性の生殖器官の形成にどのような影響を与えるのか調べた研究は非常に興味深い。

セシウム137による土壌汚染が15〜40Ci/km^{2}と、常に放射性物質にさらされる環境で生活している少女たちがいる。この少女たちの体内の女性生殖器官は発育が遅れていた。調査を受けた少女たちの37％で二次性徴の発現が遅れ、81％の少女たちで月経周期の異常がみられた。脳下垂体性腺刺激ホルモンの分泌機能異常が39％の少女たちに指摘された。31.5％の症例ではステロイドホルモンの産生障害（糖質コルチコイドホルモンの生合成の障害）も指摘された。調査の結果は、放射能汚染地域に住む少女たちに内分泌機能の低下があることを明らかにした。さらに、生殖機能の調節障害も示された。

性成熟の障害の程度と放射線の被曝量のあいだには相関があることが明らかにされている[32]。この知見は、動物実験でも確認された。エサを通じて妊娠中の母親の体内にセシウム137が取り込まれると、仔の生殖器官の発育が障害される。具体的には、セシウム137で体内汚染された母親から生まれた仔の卵巣では、思春期に成熟卵胞が統計的に有意に少なくなっており、閉鎖卵胞は対照よりも増えていることが明らかになった。その実験動物の仔の卵巣では、成熟卵胞と機能中の黄体が並存していた。さらに、卵管と子宮の粘膜の形成にも遅れが生じていた。

1.3 放射性セシウムが体内に取り込まれた状況での男性生殖器官の変化

残念ながら、体内に取り込まれたセシウム 137 が、男性の生殖器官にどのような影響を与えるのか、十分な医学的情報はない。他方、体外からの電離放射線照射が男性生殖器官に与える影響については詳細に研究されている。

雄性生殖細胞は、電離放射線によって傷つけられやすい。150 ミリシーベルト（mSv）の比較的弱い放射線照射でも、一過性の無精子症が起きる可能性がある。6 Sv 以上の放射線を一度に照射すれば、すべての雄が完全な不妊症となる。

雄性生殖細胞の放射線感受性は、放射線照射時の細胞増殖の勢いと細胞分化の程度によって異なる。電離放射線の照射に対して、増殖中の精原細胞は極めて傷つけられやすい。一方、精母細胞の電離放射線に対する感受性は精原細胞よりは低く、精子形成細胞の感受性はずっと低い（図 1.3.1）。

精子幹細胞が生存能力を失っていなければ、放射線照射後でも精子形成能力はある程度まで回復する可能性もある。

放射線照射後の男性の受精させる能力と、放射線照射した男性の子孫の状態を数世代にわたって観察すること。以上のふたつが、放射線照射が男性生殖器官に与える影響を評価するうえでの主な判定基準となることを強調しておく。

3 グレイ（Gy）の放射線を雄ラットに照射した後、長期間観察すると（1、3、6 カ月）、精巣上体中の精子数が減少し、精巣中の核酸と蛋白質の量も減っていた。この実験では、放射線照射したオスの受精させる能力も大幅に減退した[12]。V・N・ゾロツヒナとV・G・ブツの研究では、1 日 25 ラドずつ 3 日間、合わせて 75 ラドの放射線を雄ラットの全身に照射した[19]。A・I・グラドコフらの研究では、雄ラットに 0.25 Gy と 0.75 Gy のエックス線を照射した[15]。それらの結果でも、放射線照射された雄ラットは受精させる能力が大幅に減退した。A・I・グラドコフらの実験では、異常な配偶子の数が増加したことが注目される[15]。

精原細胞や精子幹細胞の段階で、0.1 〜 1.0 Gy の放射線を雄マウスに照射した実験がある[24]。この実験では VAαVC と SVA 系のマウスが使用された。雄マウスに放射線を照射した後で雌マウスと交配させたところ、子宮に着床

図 1.3.1 精子形成の模式図

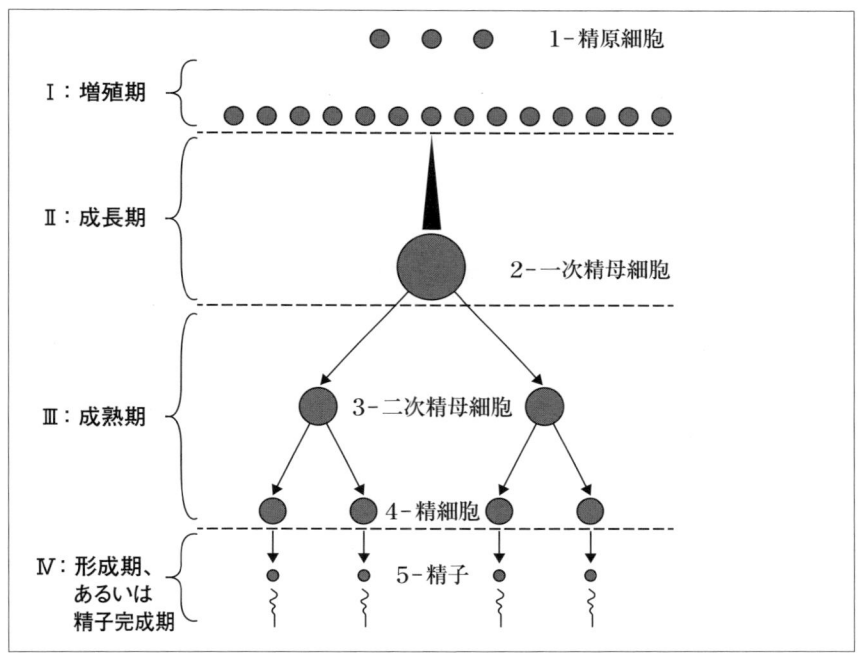

する前に胚子が死亡することが多くなった [24]。

　男性機能と精子の形成は複数のホルモンによって調節されている。男性の受精させる能力は主にこれらのホルモンの産生と関連している。下垂体性濾胞刺激ホルモン（ＦＳＨ）は精子分泌上皮に作用する。ライディッヒ細胞のテストステロン分泌は黄体形成ホルモン（ＬＨ）によって刺激を受ける。睾丸の内分泌部は、これらの性腺刺激ホルモンによって制御されている。

　テストステロンは精子幹細胞に直接作用してその状態を変化させる。ＦＳＨは精原細胞の有糸分裂を促進し、精子形成の完成も促進する。

　性ホルモンの産生は、外部放射線被曝や内部被曝の影響で減少することが示されている [3, 6, 9]。発育中の生殖器官は、放射線被曝によって非常に傷つけられやすい。この点から、グロドノ医科大学のおこなった研究は興味深い [38]。その研究では出生前と出生後の発育過程で、実験動物にセシウム 137 が投与された。その結果、セシウム 137 は雄の生殖器官の形成に悪影響を与えた。そして、テストステロンの産生と精子の形成が障害されることが明らかにな

った[38]。

セシウム 137 は生殖細胞を直接的に障害し、生殖細胞の構造や機能を変化させる。しかしそれ以外に、生殖細胞のゲノム構造も変化させることを考慮する必要がある。

1.4 放射性セシウムがもたらす突然変異誘発作用

体重1gあたり27kBqのセシウム137を雄ラットに経口的に一度に投与した。すると、投与210日から230日後に、雄ラットの生殖細胞内で一価染色体と染色体断片が統計的に有意に増加した。このセシウム137を投与した雄ラットを正常な雌ラットと交配させた。すると、子宮着床前と着床後の両方で子宮内での胎児の死亡が増加した[13]。この研究者たちはセシウム137を投与した雄ラットの体内で、ゲノムに病的な変化が起きたことが影響して胎児の死亡が増加したと考えている。

CC57W/MY系のマウスの雌を用いた生殖機能の研究でも同様な結果が得られた。マウスたちは2世代にわたってチェルノブイリとキエフの動物施設で飼育されていた。チェルノブイリの動物飼育施設にいた雌マウスを正常な雄マウスと交配させた。すると、正常な雌マウスと交配させた場合と比較して、同腹仔と新生仔の数が20〜30%減少しており、胚子の子宮着床前の死亡も増加していた[27]。

チェルノブイリ原発から30km圏内に棲息しているラットの子孫では、骨髄細胞の染色体に構造異常が高い頻度でみられた。間質性欠失と他の2ヒット染色体異常の形態（二動原体染色体、環状染色体、染色体転座）が記録されている[20]。

R・I・ゴンチャロワとN・I・リャボコニの研究では、放射性物質の汚染地域で育てた食物を実験用の雄マウスに与えて飼育した。すると、雄マウスの体内では放射性セシウム濃度が853Bq/kgと1103Bq/kgに達した。その結果、雄マウスの生殖細胞と骨髄細胞では染色体とゲノムの突然変異が増加した[16, 17]。

チェルノブイリ原発事故の後、同様の研究が住民を対象にして何年間もお

こなわれた。しかし、そうした調査では科学的に有意差を認める結果は得られなかった。住民を対象とした研究の多くでは、メンデルの遺伝法則にしたがう遺伝性の病気や多因子性の先天性奇形の発生頻度に、体内に取り込まれた放射性セシウムの影響が現れたということはできなかった[11, 21, 23]。

セシウム137で汚染されたゴメリ州の郡部に7～8年のあいだ居住した後、ミンスク市に移住してきた子どもたちの末梢血のリンパ球では、二動原体染色体と環状染色体の形態をとる染色体異常の頻度が高かったことが確認されている。これらの染色体異常は、放射線被曝によって起きる不安定型染色体異常の指標として知られている[1, 11, 35]。

チェルノブイリ原発事故の非常事態が収拾した後、発育奇形の数がベラルーシ全土で急激に増えてきた。その増加分には多発性発育奇形、手足の縮小奇形、多指症の頻度の増大が大きく寄与している。これらの発育奇形には新規の優性突然変異が大きく関与している。

単発性や多発性の先天性奇形の発生率の分析結果から、土壌汚染が15Ci/km^{2}の郡では、1997～1998年のあいだに生まれた子どもたちの奇形発生率が対照郡より高いことが示された[36, 37]。汚染地域で奇形発生率が上がったことを認めたこれらの報告では、セシウム137による土壌汚染と人びとが受けた平均被曝量しか検討されておらず、両親や子どもたちの体内に取り込まれたセシウム137による、実際の体内被曝量は考慮されていない。たとえ同じ村内でも、住民の社会的、経済的な状況、教育水準、口にする食物の違いによって、体内の放射性セシウム濃度に大きなばらつきがあることを述べておく必要がある。ヒリチフ村とニロフ村で1986年と1987年に生まれた子どもたちのあいだでは、体内のセシウム137とセシウム134濃度が、上は1773.6Bq/kg、下は69.8Bq/kgの範囲にまで広がって大きなばらつきがあった。当然、その子どもたちのあいだでは、体内の放射性セシウムによる被曝の負荷量は大きく異なっていた。

1.5 妊娠中および授乳期間中における放射性核種の体内取り込みの特徴

　放射性セシウムの体内への蓄積過程は複雑で、今日でもいまだに十分な研究がなされていない。著者らは以前、体内の放射性セシウム濃度が、性別や年齢、体の生理的状態、臓器や組織の構造や代謝の性質、さらに Rh 式赤血球表面抗原によっても影響を受けることを明らかにした[3, 5, 7]。具体的には同一のエサを与えても、雌の方が雄より体内の放射性セシウム濃度が低くなる（図 1.5.1）。

　しかし、妊娠は特殊な生理状態であり、母親の消化管で放射性セシウムが多量に吸収される。哺乳類では動物でもヒトでも、放射性セシウムの大部分は、胎盤で吸収されてしまい、胎児の体内にはほとんど取り込まれない（図 1.5.2）。しかし、妊娠中の病気や胎児の発育によっては、発育中の胎児の臓器で放射性セシウムの濃度が非常に高くなることもあり得る[6, 8]。

　ヒトや多くの動物の胎盤にみられる血絨毛型の構造が、放射性セシウムの胎盤内貯留に寄与しているかもしれない。放射性セシウムは、授乳期間中に母乳を介して母親から仔の体内に入り込む。この場合、母親の体からは放射性セシウムが取り除かれ、母体の放射性セシウム濃度は低下する。しかし同時に、仔の体内では放射性セシウム濃度が上昇してゆく[5, 56]。

　この点から、白ラットによる動物実験の結果は注目に値する。妊娠中の第 10 日目から 15 日目まで、白ラットの胃の中に 5 ml のセシウム 137 水溶液を連日投与した。対照群の白ラットには妊娠中の同じ時期に、生理的食塩水を毎日 5 ml 投与した。実験群の白ラットは 19 匹で、対照群の白ラットは 23 匹だった。実験群の白ラットからは 152 匹の仔ラットが、対照群からは 224 匹の仔ラットが生まれた。それらの仔ラットを観察し、仔ラットの体内の放射性セシウム濃度も記録した。実験群の白ラットと対照群の白ラットにはまったく同じ量のエサを与え、同一の環境で飼育したことを強調しておく。

　表 1.5.1 に放射分析の結果を示した。妊娠期間中の第 10 日から 15 日目までセシウム 137 を投与すると、分娩直後の第 1 日目には母親ラット体内のセシウム 137 濃度が 128.70 ± 6.52Bq/kg となった。その一方で、仔ラットでは体内のセシウム 137 濃度が 36.6 ± 7.46Bq/kg にとどまり、母親ラットよりも統計的に有意に低かった。分娩後とその後の授乳期間中に母親ラットと仔ラッ

図 1.5.1　動物実験の雌と雄の体内のセシウム 137 濃度

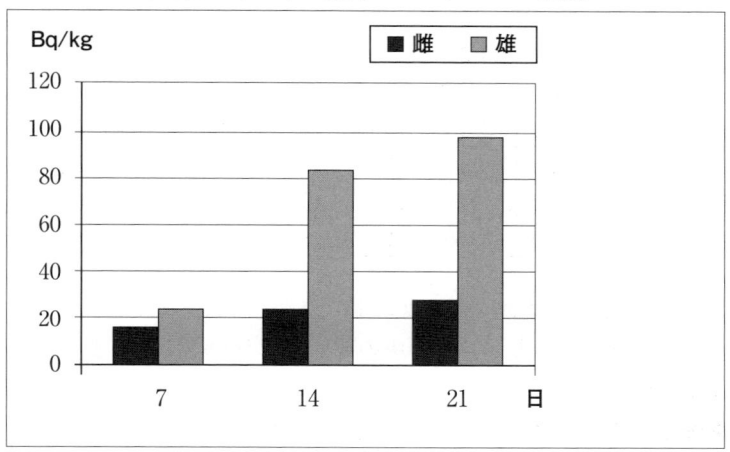

図 1.5.2　哺乳期中の実験群の母親と仔の体内のセシウム 137 濃度の変遷

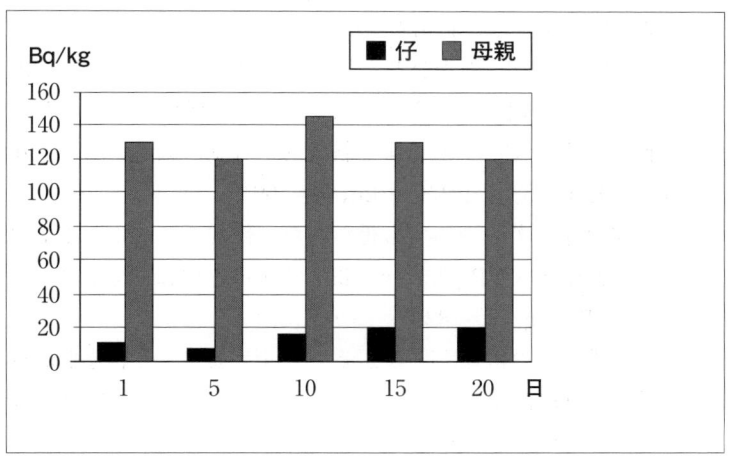

トの両方で、体内のセシウム 137 濃度はどんどん低下した。分娩後 10 日目と 20 日目には、実験群の仔ラットでは体内の放射性セシウム濃度が、対照群の仔ラットと同程度になった。

しかし、分娩 20 日目以降に仔ラットが自分でエサをとるようになると、実験群の仔ラットでは、体内のセシウム 137 保有量が増加し、対照群の仔ラットよりもはっきりと高くなった。

表 1.5.1　母親ラットと仔ラットの体内セシウム 137 濃度

(Bq/kg)

分娩後の日数	実験ラット群		対照ラット群	
	母親ラット	仔ラット	母親ラット	仔ラット
第 1 日目	128.30 ± 6.52	36.64 ± 7.46	12.10 ± 7.59	3.95 ± 1.00
第 10 日目	34.46 ± 10.44	7.80 ± 1.53	8.53 ± 1.73	4.29 ± 1.36
第 20 日目	22.06 ± 6.23	9.69 ± 4.05	10.95 ± 4.20	6.29 ± 2.88
第 30 日目	19.32 ± 4.34	35.55 ± 5.92	18.74 ± 4.01	16.71 ± 2.49

　このように、子宮内で発育期にセシウム 137 の影響を受けた仔ラットは、自分でエサをとるようになると、エサの中の放射性セシウムをより多く体内に取り込むようになる。

　この事実を確認するためには、もっと研究が必要である。しかしこの結果は、分娩後の生存にとって、子宮内での発育期がほかにないほどの重要性を持っていることを示している。

　胎盤内のセシウム 137 蓄積量は、胎児の性別で違いを認めなかった[39]。

　血液型が Rh$^+$ の人びとは、Rh$^-$ の人びとよりも放射性セシウムを多く体内に取り込むことが、著者らの研究で明らかになった[5]。胎盤の放射性セシウム濃度も Rh$^-$ の女性のほうが、Rh$^+$ の女性より統計的に有意に低かった（88.76 ± 12.37Bq/kg、$n=41$ 対 137.53 ± 12.98Bq/kg、$n=169$）

　同様の結果が、ゴメリ市の若者たちでも得られた。体内のセシウム 137 濃度は Rh$^-$ の人びとで 18.09 ± 3.88Bq/kg（$n=43$）であったのに対し、Rh$^+$ の人びとでは 23.81 ± 8.22Bq/kg（$n=182$）と高かった。

　放射性セシウムの膜構造への結合に関する研究[25]を考慮すると、赤血球表面に Rh 因子を提示する抗原決定基が、体内への放射性セシウムの取り込み過程に関与している可能性が考えられる。

1.6 放射性セシウムの体内取り込みにともなう出生前と出生後の発育の病理

1.6.1 体内に取り込まれたセシウム137量を考慮したヒトの先天性障害の評価

チェルノブイリ原発事故の後に、先天性発育障害がゴメリ州だけでなくベラルーシ全体で増えたとする科学的報告はある[11, 21, 23]。しかし、奇形の発生に、体内に取り込まれた放射性セシウムがはたす役割についてはまったく考慮されなかった。しかし、放射能汚染地帯に住む母親から得られた胎児では、肺の異形成を中心とした組織中に放射性セシウムの存在が記録された[26]。

ゴメリ州の医療施設で、医療上の必要性によって15週から25週の妊娠期間で中絶した先天性発育障害のある胎児とその胎盤を放射分析した。その結果、胎児と胎盤の中にセシウム137が存在することが明らかになった。放射分析の結果、胎盤のセシウム137濃度は、胎児のそれより高かった。胎盤のセシウム137濃度は61.50 ± 13.50Bq/kg、胎児のそれは25.40 ± 3.20Bq/kgであった。

中枢神経系の先天性障害のある胎児では、胎盤の放射性セシウム濃度がずっと高かった（85.40 ± 32.70Bq/kg）。多くは先天性発育障害のある胎児を研究の対象としたことを述べておく。この先天性発育障害は、多因子性要因、つまり遺伝性の要因と外部の要因の影響が重なり合って発生すると考えられている[22]。中枢神経系の先天性奇形ではとくに無脳症と囊胞性二分脊椎が多くみられた（42例中の16例）。

妊娠中にゴメリ州に住んでいた母親から生まれ、分娩当日に死亡した子どもでは、内臓にセシウム137が非常に多く蓄積していたことが記録されている。この子どもでは、心臓、腎臓、肝臓、甲状腺の実質細胞に顕著な変性と変性壊死があることが組織学的検査で指摘された。以下の症例も、この結論を支持するものである。

【症例１】 男児Ａは出生時体重950g、身長38cm。分娩後３日と20分で死亡。
　臨床診断：子宮内感染症。多臓器不全。早産。
　病理解剖診断：原因不明の子宮内敗血症。肺の組織構造、脳、腎臓の形態学的な未成熟。無気肺。脳浮腫。急性腎不全。臓器の実質変性。全身的な静脈鬱血。早産。出生時の著しい低体重。

表1.6.1に臓器のセシウム137濃度を示す。

【症例２】 女児Ｄは出生時体重750g、身長34cm。分娩後40分で死亡。
　臨床診断：肺疾患。多臓器不全。早産。出生時の著しい低体重。
　病理解剖診断：肺疾患（無気肺）。肺、脳、腎臓の組織構造の形態的未成熟。脳浮腫。内臓の実質変性。全身的な静脈鬱血。漿膜下出血。早産。出生時の著しい低体重。

表1.6.2に臓器のセシウム137濃度を示す。

【症例３】 男児Ｖは出生時体重3500g、身長51cm。分娩後５カ月と12日で死亡。
　臨床診断：混合病因による腸性敗血症（ネズミチフス菌＋黄色ブドウ球菌）、膿敗血症型（両側性融合性巣状気管支肺炎、右側胸膜炎、急性小腸結腸炎）。劇症の臨床経過。敗血症性ショック。多臓器不全。免疫不全状態。急性ウィルス性呼吸器感染症。滲出性カタル性体質。Ⅱ型のくる病、亜急性の臨床経過。混合病因による貧血、中等度。
　病理解剖診断：混合細菌性病因による敗血症（黄色ブドウ球菌＋ネズミチフス菌Ａ型 細菌型386 － 389番）、カタル性腸炎、剥離性肺炎、巣状漿液性間質性心筋炎、肝炎、腎炎、脾腫。溶血性尿毒症症候群。両側性漿液線維素性胸膜炎。脳浮腫。肝細胞の顆粒状変性と脂肪変性。腎尿細管上皮の顆粒状変性と壊死。全身性の静脈鬱血、血管内にフィブリン血栓と塞栓；漿膜下出血。限局性結節性唾液腺炎。

表1.6.3に臓器のセシウム濃度を示す。

【症例４】 男児Ａは出生時体重1690g、身長42cm。分娩後３日と５時間で死亡。

臨床診断：肺疾患。脳内出血。右側気胸。多臓器不全。早産。
病理解剖診断：大脳側脳室内のタンポナーデ（凝血塊）を伴う大量の両側性脳室内出血、肺疾患と無気肺、ヒアリン膜。右側の気胸。脳浮腫。内臓の実質変性。

表1.6.4に臓器のセシウム137濃度を示す。

【症例5】男児Kは出生時体重3200g、身長52cm。分娩後10日と2時間で死亡。
臨床診断：多発性の先天性奇形、肺鬱血を伴う先天性心疾患、両側性の硬口蓋軟口蓋裂、胎生発育不全の徴候（ルビンスタイン－テイビ症候群）。両側性の大葉性気管支肺炎、急性の臨床経過、Ⅲ度の呼吸不全。直接ビリルビン優位性黄疸。
病理解剖診断：多発性の先天性奇形。心室中隔欠損、両側性水腎症、両側性完全貫通性口蓋裂。播種性血管内凝固症候群、壊死巣を伴う両側性多分画性線維素膿性出血性肺炎。脳浮腫。

表1.6.5に臓器のセシウム137濃度を示す。

【症例6】女児Yは出生時体重3970g、身長55cm。分娩後9時間10分で死亡。
臨床診断：子宮内感染症。多臓器不全。
病理解剖診断：子宮内感染症（ヘルペス）、先天性肺疾患、胸膜炎、間質性肝炎、膵臓間質への巣状細胞浸潤、腎臓、上皮の腫脹、肺細胞、神経細胞、肝細胞、腎尿細管上皮の過染色性と核内封入体。全身性静脈鬱血。内臓の実質変性。低酸素脳症。

表1.6.6に臓器のセシウム137濃度を示す。

上記の症例は、死亡した子どもたちの臓器にセシウム137が非常に高い濃度で蓄積していることを示している。臨床診断と病理解剖診断は、公的な医療記録に書かれている形式で提示した。先天性奇形の子どもたちの死因として、病理学者たちはさまざまな病気を挙げている。しかし著者らは、この子どもたちの本当の死亡原因は、子宮内の発育期間と出生後に受けた放射性セ

表 1.6.1　臓器のセシウム 137 濃度

臓　器	セシウム 137 濃度 (Bq/kg)
心臓	5333
肝臓	250
肺	1125
腎臓	1500
脳組織	3000
甲状腺	4333
胸腺	3000
小腸	2500
大腸	3250
胃	3750
脾臓	3500
副腎	1750
膵臓	11000

表 1.6.2　臓器のセシウム 137 濃度

臓　器	セシウム 137 濃度 (Bq/kg)
心臓	4250
肝臓	277
肺	2666
腎臓	1687
脳組織	1363
甲状腺	6250
胸腺	3833
小腸	1375
大腸	3125
胃	1250
脾臓	1500
副腎	2500
膵臓	12500

表 1.6.3　臓器のセシウム 137 濃度

臓　器	セシウム 137 濃度 (Bq/kg)
心臓	625
肝臓	525
肺	400
腎臓	250
脳組織	305
甲状腺	250
胸腺	1142
小腸	571
大腸	261
胃	1500
脾臓	428
膵臓	1312

表 1.6.4　臓器のセシウム 137 濃度

臓　器	セシウム 137 濃度 (Bq/kg)
心臓	4166
肝臓	851
肺	1195
腎臓	2250
脳組織	90
甲状腺	1900
胸腺	3833
小腸	3529
大腸	3040
脾臓	1036
副腎	2500

表 1.6.5　臓器のセシウム 137 濃度

臓　　器	セシウム 137 濃度 (Bq/kg)
心臓	1071
肝臓	882
肺	1500
腎臓	812
脳組織	1693
胸腺	714
小腸	2200
大腸	4000
脾臓	2000
副腎	4750

表 1.6.6　臓器のセシウム 137 濃度

臓　　器	セシウム 137 濃度 (Bq/kg)
心臓	1491
肝臓	1000
肺	2610
腎臓	583
脳組織	714
甲状腺	1583
胸腺	833
小腸	590
脾臓	2125
副腎	2619
膵臓	2941

シウムのもたらす毒作用であったと自信を持っていえる。

　放射分析の結果から、これらの症例は胎児と新生児に起きた放射能毒性症候群として語るのがふさわしいと考える。ウィルス学的、細菌学的検査をせずに子宮内感染症の診断をつけることが不可能なように、臓器の放射分析をせずに放射能汚染地域の胎児と新生児の真の死因を見出すことは不可能である。

1.6.2　妊娠中に放射性セシウムを体内に取り込んだ実験動物での胚胎児発生

a）白ラットでの実験

　エサに放射性セシウムをまぜ、雑種の白ラットに与えて体内に放射性セシウムを取り込ませ、その結果起きる、胚子や胎児の形態学的、機能的変化を詳細に調べることがこの研究の目的である[48]。

　実験には、妊娠した雑種雌白ラットを 137 匹、ラットの胎児を 745 匹、仔ラットを 344 匹用いた。膣内容物塗抹標本で精子を検出した日を妊娠第 1 日目とみなした。子宮内発育の第 20 日目まで、つまり分娩予定の 1 日前までの胎児を研究の対象とした。ラットの飼育と給餌は、飼育ケースの中でおこなった。セシウム 137 濃度が 5587Bq/kg の肉をエサの構成成分として毎日与え

表 1.6.7　実験に用いた母親ラット、ラットの胎児、仔ラットの数

グループ名	胚子胎児発生 数		生後発育 数	
	母親ラット	ラットの胎児	母親ラット	仔ラット
第1実験群	20	115	4	69
第1対照群	23	100	10	37
第2実験群	24	292	15	127
第2対照群	24	238	17	111
合計	91	745	46	344

たラットを第1実験群とした。セシウム137濃度が445.7Bq/kgの穀物をエサの構成成分として毎日与えたラットを第2実験群とした。放射性セシウム濃度が49.0Bq/kgの肉を含むエサを与えたラットを、第1対照群とした。放射性セシウム濃度が44.2 Bq/kgの穀物を含むエサを与えたラットを第2対照群とした。

エサの消費量から計算して、第1実験群のラットは肉からセシウム137を毎日84Bq、第1対照群は肉からセシウム137を毎日0.74Bq、第2実験群は穀物からセシウム137を毎日16Bq、第2対照群はセシウム137を毎日0.016Bq摂取したことになる。

第1実験群と第1対照群のラットでは、体内のセシウム137濃度の測定をしなかった。

第2実験群の雌ラットでは、妊娠末期に体内のセシウム137濃度が132.77 ± 10.77Bq/kgに達した。一方、第2対照群の雌ラットでは体内のセシウム137濃度が9.22 ± 2.90Bq/kgにとどまった。

実験群の雌ラットから生まれた仔ラットの体内の放射性セシウム濃度は6.47 ± 2.18Bq/kgであった。一方、対照群の雌ラットから産まれた仔ラットの体内の放射性セシウム濃度は1.61 ± 0.87Bq/kgであった。

表1.6.7に実験に用いた母親ラット、ラットの胎児、仔ラットの数を示す。

胚子胎児発生の病理を研究するため、実験群と対照群の母親ラットは妊娠第20日目にエーテル麻酔で安楽死させた後、断頭した。ラットの胎児を子宮から摘出し、発育障害を識別するため、外観を観察して体重も測定した。同腹仔のうち、ラットの胎児を1匹、ブアン固定液で固定し、残りの胎児は96°のアルコールで固定した。子宮の着床部位の数、子宮内で生きていたラット

胎児の数、母親ラット卵巣中の黄体数を数えて、子宮着床前と子宮着床後の胚子と胎児の死亡数の指標を計算した。

この研究では以下の検討をした。

1) A・P・ドイバンの修正ウィルソン法[18]を用いてラット胎児の臓器の状態を検討。この目的のため、ブアン固定液で固定したラットの胎児をパラフィン包埋し、カミソリの刃を用いて連続平行切片を作成した。

2) ラットの胎児の骨格骨の状態の検討。この目的のため、96°のアルコールで固定したラットの胎児はA・P・ドイバンの修正ドーソン法で処理し、アリザリンレッドで骨化標識部位を染色した[18]。ラットの胎児の骨格長（頭頂－尾骨長）をコンパスで測定した。個別の骨の骨化標識の長さは接眼マイクロメーター、双眼拡大鏡 MBS-10 を用いて測定した。

3) 妊娠第 20 日目に、第 1 実験群と第 2 実験群の雌ラットの血液中の総ビリルビン、尿素、クレアチニン、総蛋白、リン、トリグリセリド、コレステロール、アルブミン、グルコース、アルカリフォスファターゼ活性、アラニンアミノトランスフェラーゼ、アスパラギン酸アミノトランスフェラーゼを、ベックマン社製シンクロン CX 分析器を用いて測定した。

スチューデントの t 検定に従う統計的変法で、得られた結果を検定した。

実験結果から、放射性セシウム濃度が 5587Bq/kg の肉を含むエサを妊娠第 1 日目から与えた第 1 実験群の雌の白ラットでは、胚子の子宮着床前の死亡が、対照群よりも有意に多いことが明らかになった（2.27 ± 0.52 対 0.80 ± 0.31、$p < 0.05$）。放射性セシウム濃度が 445.7Bq/kg の燕麦をエサとして与えた第 2 実験群の妊娠した雌ラットでは、胚子の子宮着床前死亡の統計的に有意な増加はみられなかった。ラット胎児の子宮着床後の死亡率では、実験群と対照群のあいだで違いを認めなかった。実験群のラット胎児では、骨格骨の平均長が対応する対照群のラット胎児よりも統計的に有意に短かった（表 1.6.8）。

中手骨と中足骨の骨化中心が欠如しているラットの胎児数は、対照群よりも第 1 実験群と第 2 実験群で多かった。

骨格骨の状態を調べた結果、第 1 実験群のラットの胎児では、すべての骨

表 1.6.8　実験群のラットの胎児の骨格系の指標

指標名	第1実験群	第1対照群	第2実験群	第2対照群
骨格の長さ (mm)	21.39 ± 0.48	24.70 ± 0.41	23.84 ± 0.39	25.55 ± 0.31
中手骨と中足骨の骨化中心を欠く胎児の比率 (%)	31.4	13.0	33.8	25.0

格骨で左右対称の骨化標識部位の低形成がみられた。さらに、恥骨の骨化標識部位の両側性の欠如や、第二、第四中手骨と、第二、第三、第四中足骨の骨化中心の欠如もみられた。

　第2実験群のラットの胎児の骨格骨の検討をした。第四中手骨と第二、第三中足骨の骨化標識部位の長さは、第2実験群と対応する対照群とのあいだで有意差を認めなかった。しかし、それ以外のすべての骨格骨で、骨化標識部位の長さは左右とも統計的に有意に短くなっていた。また第2実験群のラット胎児では、恥骨の両側の骨化標識部位の欠如、両側の第二中手骨、第四中足骨の骨化標識部位に欠如がみられた。

　第1実験群のラット胎児では、上腕骨の骨化標識部位の長さが対照群と比べて20〜25％短縮していた。大腿骨では30％、坐骨では55〜60％短縮していた。第2実験群のラット胎児でも、上腕骨の骨化標識部位の長さが対照群と比べて16〜20％短縮し、大腿骨では25〜27％短縮、坐骨では43〜54％短縮していた。

　第2実験群の母親ラットでは、対照群と比較して、妊娠第20日目に血清アルブミン濃度が上昇していた（13.83 ± 1.11g/l 対 10.50 ± 0.93g/l、$p<0.05$）、さらに血清カルシウム濃度も上昇していた（1.87 ± 0.18mmol/l 対 1.31 ± 0.16mmol/l、$p<0.05$）。それ以外の検査した代謝指標には、実験群と対照群の間に有意差を認めなかった。

　ビスター系の雌ラットに妊娠期間の後半の妊娠第10〜第15日目まで、セシウム137の水溶液を与えたところ、出産した仔ラットでは体内のセシウム137濃度が対照群に比べ有意に高かった（36.64 ± 7.46Bq/kg、$n=152$ 対 3.95 ± 1.00Bq/kg、$n=224$）。生まれた仔ラットの臓器には病的変化がみられた。仔ラットの心臓には、線維間浮腫、心筋細胞の瀰漫性壊死、心筋細胞の変性がみられた。肝臓には、肝細胞の蛋白変性、ディッセ腔の拡大、肝小葉中心

図 1.6.1

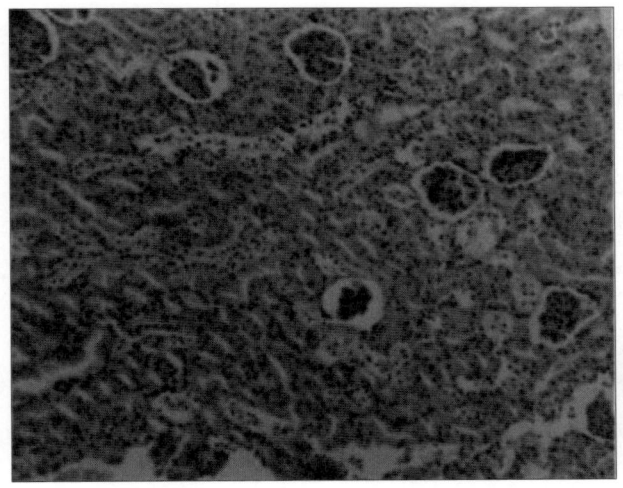

体内の放射性セシウム濃度が40Bq/kgであった、分娩直後の仔ラットの腎臓の組織構造。糸球体の萎縮と破壊、尿細管上皮の蛋白変性と壊死がみられる。ヘマトキシリンエオジン染色。125倍。

部の充血がみられた。腎臓には糸球体の破壊、輸入細動脈の攣縮、尿細管上皮の強い変性がみられた（図 1.6.1）。哺乳期間の生後第 10 日目と第 20 日目の仔ラットにも同じ変化が認められた。これらの病理変化は 30 日齢の仔ラットでとくに顕著に認められた。30 日齢の仔ラットは自分でエサを摂るようになり、放射性セシウムの体内濃度が著しく高かった（表 1.5.1）。

このように、セシウム 137 が妊娠中の母親ラットの体内に入り込むと、胚子と胎児の発育過程が著しく障害され、子宮粘膜への着床段階での胚子の死亡として現れる。さらに、ラットの胎児の骨組織には、大部分の骨格骨の骨化標識部位の低形成という形態をとる病理変化が起こる。またラットの胎児の臓器の細胞には変性と変性壊死が起きる。

b）シリアンハムスターでの実験

この研究では、妊娠中のシリアンハムスターの雌にセシウム 137 を投与し、セシウム 137 が胎児の発育に与える影響を調べた。

体重が 100〜150g の妊娠中のシリアンハムスターの雌を 29 匹使用した。膣内容塗抹標本に精子が存在したときを受精時とした。そのうち 18 匹には、妊娠第 6 日目と第 8 日目、100Bq の放射活性のセシウム 137 が入った滅菌水溶液 1ml を腹腔内に注射し、これを実験群とした。残りの 11 匹には、妊娠

第6日目と第8日目に1mlの生理的食塩水を腹腔内に注射し、これを対照群とした。実験群と対照群の母親シリアンハムスターの体内セシウム137濃度は、RUG-2放射計を用いて妊娠第10日目に記録した。

分娩予定日前日の妊娠第15日目に、シリアンハムスターの胎児の状態を調べた。この実験でも、母親シリアンハムスターの卵巣内の黄体の数と子宮内着床部位の数を数えた。

それをもとに、子宮着床前、および子宮着床後の胚子と胎児の死亡率を計算した。シリアンハムスターの胎児と胎盤の重さも計測した。胎盤の重さは、胎児の重さと比較し、胎盤－胎児係数という形で評価した。ハムスターの胎児は、肉眼的に観察できる身体構造の大きな欠陥（先天性奇形）を識別するため、外観を観察したあと、ブワン固定液か96°のアルコールに入れた。ブワン固定液で固定された胎児は、ウィルソン－ドイバン法[18]で臓器の状態を検討した。96°のアルコールで固定された胎児はドーソン法で処理し、骨格骨はアリザリンレッドで染色した[18]。以上の方法で、実験群と対照群の合わせて208匹の胎児を検討した。

この実験では、対照群の母親ハムスターの体内セシウム137濃度は4～20Bq/kgの範囲にあった（平均12.4 ± 1.7Bq/kg）。対照群の母親ハムスター全11匹のうち、5匹の母親ハムスター（妊娠例の46％）から得た胎児には、先天性奇形（外脳症、頭蓋脳ヘルニア、口唇口蓋裂、無眼球症、小眼球症）がみられた。上記の先天性奇形は、多因子性グループに属している。多因子性先天性奇形の発症は、両親が遺伝性素因を持っているか否かという問題と、妊娠中の環境因子の影響に依存すると考えられている[22]。子宮内発育の第15日目に胎児を検査したが、対照群の母親ハムスターから得た101匹の胎児では、そのうちの20匹（20％）の胎児にしか、前述の先天性奇形はみられなかった。妊娠第6日目と第8日目にセシウム137を投与すると、妊娠第10日目に、母親ハムスターの体内セシウム137濃度は平均246.60 ± 20.10Bq/kgに達した。シリアンハムスターでは、妊娠第6日目から9日目は胎児の器官形成と胎盤形成の時期にあたり、胚胎児発生の臨界期のひとつである。セシウム137を投与された母親ハムスターの胎児の状態を妊娠第15日目に調べたところ、セシウム137による催奇性と胎児死亡作用をすべての妊娠例で認めた。実験群の18匹の母親ハムスターのうち9匹（50％）では、胎児の器官形成と胎盤形成の段階ですべての胎児が死亡していた。実験群の残りの9匹の母親

ハムスターにおける、母親ハムスター1匹ごとの子宮着床後の胎児の平均死亡数 5.9 ± 1.0 も示された。対照群の胎児の平均死亡数は 1.6 ± 0.4 と有意に少なかった（$p<0.01$）。実験群の母親ハムスター18匹のうち9匹（50％）の母親ハムスターでは、子宮内ですべての胎児が死亡するということはなかった。しかし、その母親ハムスターから得た胎児では、先天性奇形が指摘された。セシウム137を投与された実験群の母親ハムスターから得た全部で107匹の胎児のうち、63匹（59％）に、外脳症、頭蓋脳ヘルニア、口唇口蓋裂、小上顎症、小下顎症、小眼球症、無眼球症（図 1.6.2、1.6.3、1.6.4、1.6.5）といった先天性奇形が認められた。実験群から得た胎児の体重と対照群から得た胎児の体重には有意差を認めなかった（実験群 1.29 ± 0.04g、対照群 1.49 ± 0.10g）。実験群と対照群の比較では、胎盤－胎児係数にも有意差を認めなかった。

大変残念なことに、実験時、著者らはシリアンハムスターの胎児のような非常に軽くかつ小さなものの放射性セシウム含有量を正確に測定できる機器を持っていなかった。したがって、以下ではセシウム137濃度の最高値と最低値だけを示す。実験群のハムスターの胎児では、体内セシウム137濃度は 218〜464Bq/kg の範囲にあった。実験群の母親ハムスターの胎盤のセシウム137濃度は 511〜2250Bq/kg の範囲にあった。

子宮内ですべての胎児が死亡した妊娠例では、子宮と胎児組織のセシウム137濃度が 426〜1806Bq/kg の範囲にあった。

上記のデータは、妊娠中のシリアンハムスターの体内にセシウム137が取り込まれると、胎児の発育が著しい悪影響を受けることを示している。この場合、ヒトでよくみられる、いわゆる多因子性の先天性奇形[11]が出現する。多因子性先天性奇形は、遺伝的な欠陥と環境要因の影響が重なって発症すると信じられている[22, 23]。

放射性セシウムが比較的少量でも体内に取り込まれれば、母親－胎児系が影響を受け、多因子性先天性奇形を発症する条件が準備される。欠陥ゲノムをもっていても、その欠陥が形質発現しない場合もある。しかし、放射性セシウムが少量でも体内に取り込まれると、母親－胎児系がその影響を受け、欠陥ゲノムが形質発現しやすくなるということである。

前述の実験結果を踏まえ、体内の代謝過程は障害するが、母親ハムスターは死なない程度の濃度になるように、セシウム137の投与量を調整して実験

図 1.6.2

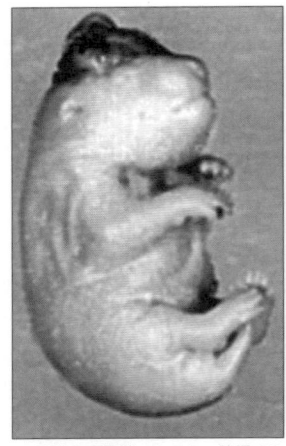

15日齢の実験群ハムスター胎児でみられた外脳症（頭蓋骨の欠如）、無眼球症（眼球の欠如）。

図 1.6.3

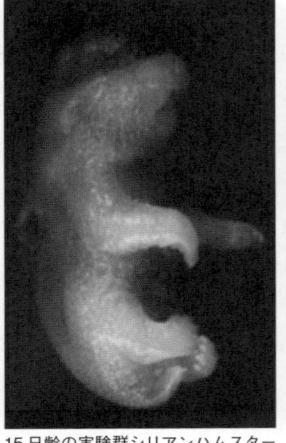

15日齢の実験群シリアンハムスター胎児にみられた外脳症（頭蓋骨の欠如）、小下顎症（下顎の低形成）、無眼球症（眼球の欠如）。

図 1.6.4

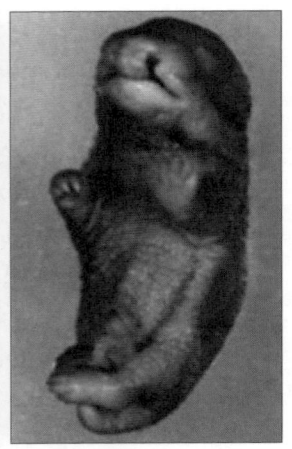

15日齢の実験群シリアンハムスター胎児にみられた両側性口唇口蓋裂。

した。そして、妊娠第6日目と第8日目の胎児の器官形成と胎盤形成の時期に、母親ハムスターにセシウム137を注射した。その実験では、特徴的な先天性奇形がすべての胎児に指摘された。セシウム137の影響で細胞がエネルギー不足に陥り、母親－胎児系に代謝障害が起きる。著者らは、その代謝障害が原因となって、シリアンハムスターの胎児に多因子起源の先天性奇形が発症すると考えている。

　白ラットでは、セシウム137が子宮内の胎児発育過程に影響しても、シリアンハムスターでみられた多因子性先天性奇形は発生しなかった。しかし、白ラットの胎児でも発育障害はみられた。白ラットの胎児でみられた発育障害は、大部分の骨格骨の骨化標識部位の低形成、臓器の細胞変性と変性壊死であった。これらはセシウム137がもたらす代謝機能の障害作用を示している。白ラットを用いた実験では、多因子性先天性奇形の胎児はごく稀にしか確認されなかった。一方、シリアンハムスターを用いた実験では、多因子性先天性奇形の胎児がつねに見出されたことは強調すべきであろう。多因子性先天性奇形の発生頻度が白ラットとシリアンハムスターで違うことに関してだけは問題が残る。

　シリアンハムスターの実験では、多因子性先天性奇形の胎児は対照群で散

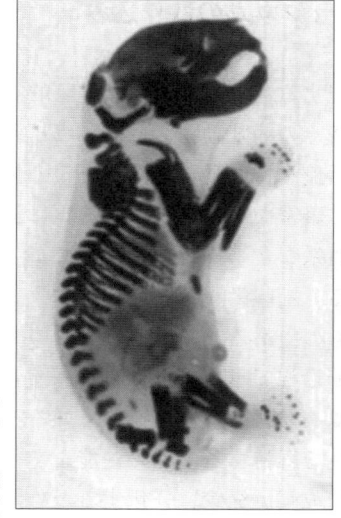

図 1.6.5

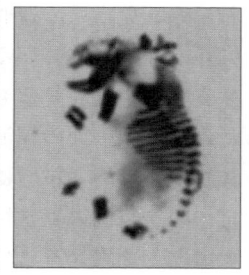

子宮内発育第 15 日目のシリアンハムスター胎児。アリザリンレッドによる骨格骨染色
  a：対照群のハムスター胎児
  b：実験群のハムスター胎児。頭蓋骨の欠如、小上顎症（上顎の低形成）、骨格骨の低形成、アリザリンレッド染色。

a   b

発的にしかみられなかった。しかし、セシウム 137 が母親－胎児系に取り込まれると多因子性先天性奇形を持つ胎児が激増した。

　このように、セシウム 137 は実験動物の胎児の発育過程に異常を引き起こす。その発育異常がどのような性質を持つかについては、胎児のゲノムの状態で決定される。胎盤の構成成分が損傷されると、胎盤の内分泌機能と免疫調節機能が障害される。このことが、胎児の奇形の形成で大きな役割を演じている可能性がある。胎盤が放射性セシウムを多量に取り込むことは確かだ。

　多因子性先天性奇形のあるヒトと動物の胎児では、胎盤で高濃度のセシウム 137 が記録された。

　以前に得られたデータ [3, 5, 6] から考えると、以下のように結論することができる。放射性セシウムが母親－胎児系に取り込まれると、代謝異常症候群とよぶべきものが起きる。そして、母親と胎児の臓器と、とくに妊娠時の一時的な器官である胎盤が、放射性セシウムによる損傷をこうむる。

1.7 胎盤の放射性セシウムの取り込み

　胎盤は妊娠時に出現するもっとも重要な一時的器官であり、胎児の発育を支えている。ヒトと多くの哺乳動物、とくにげっ歯類の胎盤は血絨毛型の構造を持つ。血絨毛型胎盤を持つ動物では、母親の体と発育中の胎児組織のあいだに血管系を介して緊密な関係が築かれる。母親と胎児の両方の内分泌系、神経系、免疫系、造血系などの重要な器官系によって母親と胎児のあいだの関係が調節されている。細胞栄養芽層と合胞体栄養細胞層の細胞は、胚外の栄養芽層を代表するものである。胎盤そのものの細胞構造と細胞間の構造は、母親と胎児の間の調節過程で重要な役割を担っている。細胞栄養芽層と合胞体栄養細胞層の細胞は高い代謝活性を持っている。この高い代謝活性のおかげで、子宮内の恒常性を維持する多くの機能を遂行することができる。胎児の臓器と組織が正常に成長、発育、分化するためには、ビタミンと微量元素が不可欠である。細胞栄養芽層と合胞体栄養細胞層の細胞は、母親から胎児へのビタミンと微量元素の移行を、ピノサイトーシス、エクソサイトーシス、あるいは拡散によって支えている [28]。

　細胞栄養芽層の細胞はプロゲステロン、エストロゲン、絨毛性ゴナドトロピン、絨毛性ソマトトロピン、絨毛性甲状腺刺激ホルモン、それに絨毛性黄体刺激ホルモンを産生する。細胞栄養芽層の細胞が胎盤の内分泌機能を担っている [28]。胎児の発育と胎盤の"老化"にともない、細胞栄養芽層の細胞は合胞体栄養細胞層に変化する。合胞体栄養細胞層も生物学的に活動的である。母親と胎児のあいだの免疫連関に対する栄養膜上皮の関与にとくに注目する必要がある。母親の免疫グロブリン、特に Ig M と Ig G の吸着が栄養膜細胞の細胞膜で起きることは証明されていると思われる [4]。

　母親の血液の細胞は栄養膜構造を通って胎児の体内に入り、また胎児の血液の細胞も母親の体内に入る。胎児の赤血球の30％は、常に母親の血液中を循環していることが証明されている。胎児のリンパ球もまた母親の血液中で記録される [4]。胎児は胎盤を介して母親から免疫担当細胞と免疫グロブリンを受け取る。著者らは、1994年に発育中の胎児の免疫系の形成に関する仮説を提出した [4]。母親の免疫担当幹細胞が胎盤障壁を通過して胎児に入り、母親と胎児の液性免疫の連関が形成されるという仮説である。

　胎盤が、放射性元素を含むさまざまな元素の輸送においてどのような働き

をしているか、ほとんど研究されていない。放射性元素や非放射性元素、ほかの物質が胎盤を通過して移動することに関しては、文献ごとに正反対の結果を示すデータが存在しており、一定の知見がない。これは、放射性セシウムについても当てはまる。白ラットを用いた動物実験では、エサを通じて母親に取り込まれたセシウム137は、胎児には限られた量しか取り込まれないことが示された[5]。

一方、妊娠第10日目から15日目まで妊娠中のラットの雌にセシウム137の水溶液を投与すると、胎児の組織中にセシウム137がより顕著に蓄積する。シリアンハムスターでは、ラットの実験で示された結果よりも多くの放射性セシウムが胎盤障壁を通過して胎児に取り込まれる。ヒトでも、放射性セシウムは胎盤障壁を通過してしまう。ヒトでは、胎児の放射性セシウム濃度よりも胎盤の放射性セシウム濃度のほうが高いことに注目する必要がある[8]。先天性奇形の胎児では、放射性セシウム濃度が著しく高い。これは、胎盤の障壁機能が低下していることを意味しているかもしれない。ヒトでは、胎盤にセシウム137が蓄積すると、胎盤の構造が著しく変化する。胎盤のセシウム137濃度が100Bq/kgを超えると、妊娠の終わりが近づくにしたがい、中間絨毛が増加し、終末絨毛が減少した。絨毛は細胞栄養芽層で覆われ、間質は粗雑で結合織の細胞が増加していた。終末絨毛と中間絨毛中で合胞体栄養細胞が密集していることが注目された。これはホルモン産生のプロセスを意味している。先天性奇形の胎児の胎盤では、絨毛間質と絨毛間腔への出血の形態をとる血液循環障害が顕著にみられ、限局性の小梗塞巣も認められた。

1.8 放射性セシウムを取り込んだ母 ― 胎児系の内分泌の相互関係

妊娠した女性の体内にセシウム137が取り込まれると、発育中の胎児で大きなホルモン分泌の変化が起きる。ゴメリ医大のスタッフは、74の分娩例で母親と胎児のホルモン状態を評価した。その74分娩例を胎盤の放射性セシウム濃度によって、以下の4群にわけた。

対照群：胎盤に放射性セシウムが存在しない
第1群：胎盤の放射性セシウム濃度が1〜99Bq/kg

第2群：100 〜 199Bq/kg

第3群：200Bq/kg 以上 [39]

　その結果、胎盤の放射性セシウム濃度が高くなると、胎児の臍帯血エストラジオール濃度が著しく低下することが示された。胎盤の放射性セシウム濃度が高くなると、胎児の臍帯血テストステロン濃度は顕著に高くなった（図1.8.1）。これらの傾向は胎児が女児の場合だけでなく、男児の場合でもみられた。

　胎盤の放射性セシウム濃度が高くなると、母親の血中エストラジオール濃度が低下した。胎児の臍帯血エストラジオール濃度に対する母親の血中エストラジオール濃度の比は、全グループの平均では 0.9 だった。胎児の臍帯血テストステロン濃度に対する母親の血中テストステロン濃度の比は、対照群では 1.89 だったが、第3群では 0.49 に低下した。胎盤のセシウム 137 濃度が高くなると、胎児の臍帯血エストラジオール濃度／テストステロン濃度比が著しく低下した。胎児の臍帯血プロゲステロン濃度は、母親の血中プロゲステロン濃度よりも有意に高かった。胎児の臍帯血プロゲステロン濃度と母親の血中プロゲステロン濃度は、対照群から第3群へと増加していく傾向がみられた。

　胎盤の放射性セシウム濃度が高くなると、母親の血中甲状腺ホルモン濃度（サイロキシンとトリヨードサイロニン濃度）が明らかに高くなった。臍帯血中の胎児のサイロキシンとトリヨードサイロニン濃度は、胎盤の放射性セシウム濃度で変化しなかった。

　胎盤の放射性セシウム濃度が高くなると、母親の血中コルチゾール濃度ははっきりと増加した。反対に、胎児の臍帯血中コルチゾール濃度は低下した（図 1.8.2）。

　このように、母親－胎児系にセシウム 137 が入り込むと、何よりもまず、発育中の胎児に顕著なホルモン濃度の変化が起きる。副腎皮質にセシウム 137 が強く取り込まれることが注目される [6, 8, 49]。セシウム 137 が取り込まれると、ミトコンドリアの酵素系に機能障害が起きる [47]。セシウム 137 が副腎皮質のホルモン産生細胞に悪影響を与えるため、男性ホルモンのテストステロンの産生が増加し、女性ホルモンのエストラジオールが減少するとも考えられる。この仮説ではまず、副腎皮質の主要なホルモンであるコルチゾールの生合成が障害される。この状況が、下垂体性副腎皮質刺激ホルモンの産生増加に拍車をかけ、副腎皮質の細胞を刺激してテストステロンの過剰産生を

図 1.8.1　胎児の臍帯血エストロゲン濃度とテストステロン濃度

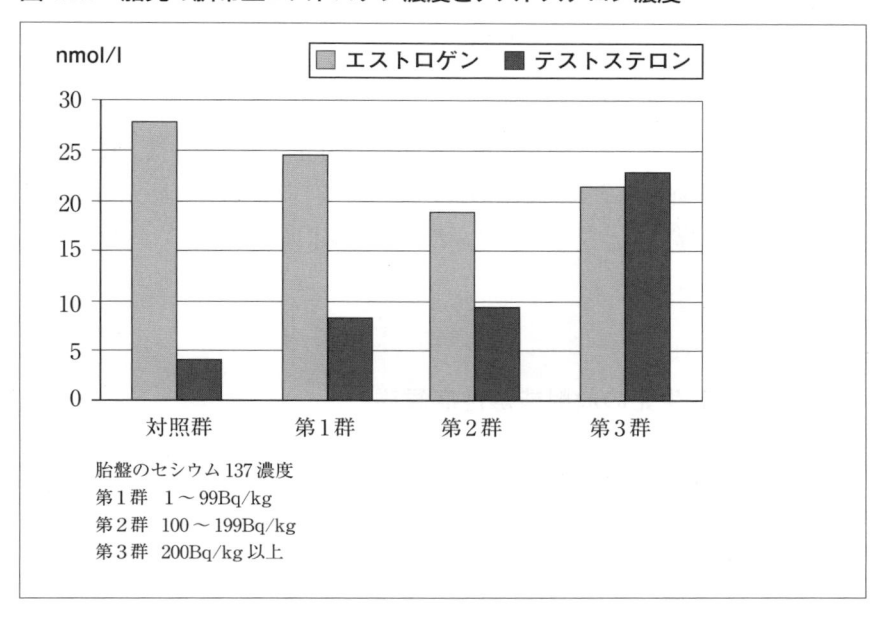

胎盤のセシウム 137 濃度
第 1 群　1〜99Bq/kg
第 2 群　100〜199Bq/kg
第 3 群　200Bq/kg 以上

図 1.8.2　実験群と対照群の母親と胎児の血中コルチゾール濃度

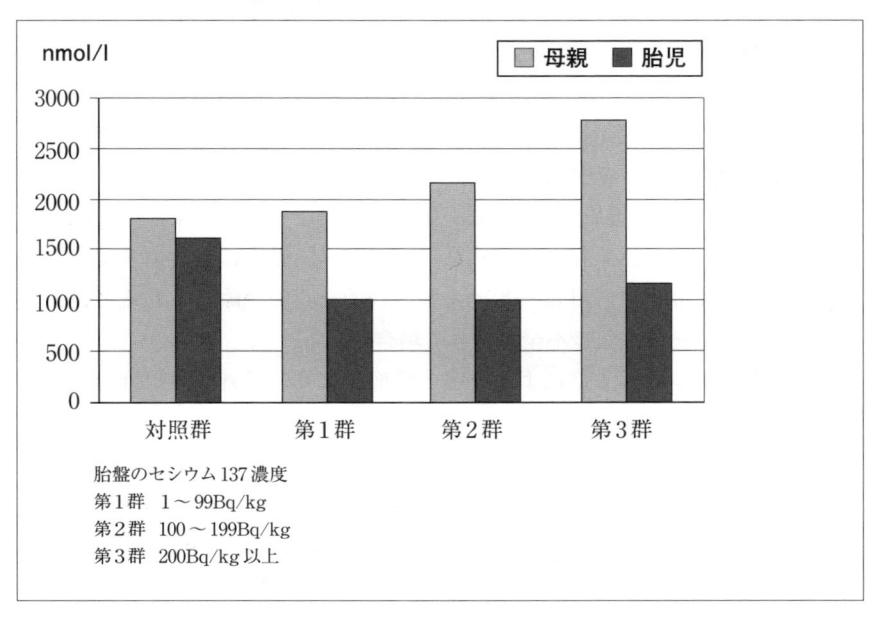

胎盤のセシウム 137 濃度
第 1 群　1〜99Bq/kg
第 2 群　100〜199Bq/kg
第 3 群　200Bq/kg 以上

招く。副腎皮質の先天性機能不全の状態が起きる。これは以後の子どもの発育過程に間違いなく悪影響を与えるだろう。放射性セシウムの影響で起きる子どもたちの内分泌状態の逆転は、子どもたちの性的発達の異常と外部環境に対する生後の適応障害を引き起こす主な原因のひとつであると著者らは考えている。そして、子どもたちが成長してから内分泌系、神経系、免疫系や、ほかの多くの器官系の病気になるのは、セシウム137の影響で胎児期からホルモン産生が異常になっていることが基礎にあると考えられる。

1.9　胎児と新生児の放射能毒性症候群

　体内に取り込まれたセシウム137は、多くの生物学的構造と、とくにある複雑な系と相互作用するようになる。それは母親−胎児系である。セシウム137が母親の体に及ぼす影響は以下の器官系の障害として現れてくる。

内分泌系：性機能の調節も含む内分泌異常。
筋肉系：生殖器の筋組織と血管壁のトーヌス（緊張度）の変化。
心血管系：子宮やほかのすべての臓器への血液供給が障害され、臓器の機能障害をともなう。
神経系：母親の神経系機能の障害は、母親と発育中の胎児のあいだの神経調節連関の異常を引き起こす。
免疫系：母親の生体防御機能が低下することで、子宮内感染症の特徴を有するウィルス感染症と細菌感染症が母親−胎児系に起きやすくなる状況をつくり出す。母親−胎児系の統合的な連関が障害されると、先天性奇形や先天性免疫不全が起きる場合がある。
泌尿器系：セシウム137による腎臓の病変により、体外へ放射性セシウムや毒素が排泄されるのが遅れ、子宮内での胎児の発育異常が起こりやすい状況をつくり出す。
造血系：セシウム137が著しく多く体内に取り込まれると、赤血球数が減少する。そして、子宮内で胎児や新生児に低酸素症が起きる。
肝胆道系：母親と胎児の代謝で重要な役割を果たしている肝臓の多くの機

能が障害される。まず、生命の維持にとって重要な物質を産生する肝臓の合成機能が障害される。さらに毒物、神経伝達物質、ホルモン、体にとって異物である環境因子を中和する能力も障害される。蛋白、脂肪、炭水化物、ミネラルの代謝の調節も障害される。肝細胞の損傷や肝細胞の脂肪変性、蛋白変性が、母親－胎児系の代謝異常を招く。

生殖系：卵巣組織、子宮、卵管の病変と、その結果起きる胎児の発育障害。

胎児の子宮内発育：放射性セシウムは胎盤に取り込まれると、胎盤の細動脈や毛細血管といった血管網や栄養膜芽層細胞と相互作用するようになる。すると、血液循環が障害され、また胎盤自体のホルモン産生が変化し、その結果として母親と胎児の内分泌系が変化する。

胎盤は、基礎的な障壁として、セシウム137が胎児の組織に入り込むことをたしかに制限するが、さまざまなことが原因となって胎盤の障壁作用が低下すると、セシウム137は胎児の組織に入り込む。そして胎児の組織を傷つけ、先天性奇形を引き起こす。

セシウム137は細胞のエネルギー産生能力を劇的に弱めてしまい、代謝の全過程を障害し、とくに蛋白分子の生合成を阻害する。このため、セシウム137が奇形の発生に関与している可能性が十分に考えられる。シリアンハムスターでの実験は、これにはっきりと当てはまる事例である。放射性セシウムの影響下では、シリアンハムスターに多くの発育障害例がみられる。それらの発育障害は多因子性先天性奇形のグループに関連する中枢神経系や、頭蓋骨の顔面部分、心臓の奇形である。多因子性先天性奇形のグループの発現は、遺伝的な欠陥の存在と、欠陥の発現を誘発する環境因子の作用に関連している[22]。突然変異が起きると一部の遺伝子では機能が失われる。つまり、突然変異により欠陥遺伝子となる。すると、染色体上で同じ位置を占める対立遺伝子群のなかの欠陥のない遺伝子が正常な表現形質を発現する安全性が確保できなくなる。つまり、ゲノムには十分なセーフティーマージンがなくなり、欠陥遺伝子が異常な表現形質を発現する可能性が高まる。このような状況で、胎児の発育過程がセシウム137によって干渉されると、異常な表現形質の発現に至る。すなわち、先天性奇形の形成に至る。このように、放射性セシウムは、親の世代では内在し形質発現しなかった遺伝的な欠陥を子どもの代で形質発現させる誘発因子として働く。

この場合、セシウム137の体内取り込み量は多くなくても胎児に異常が発現する。母親と胎児のあいだの調整関係には、免疫系、内分泌系、神経系などの調節系の関与、生合成の適正な速度の維持、表現形質の発現に必要な胎児組織の分化がある。上記のように、ゲノムに欠陥がある状況では、放射性セシウムの作用はとくに母親と胎児のあいだの調整関係の破壊に向かうと著者らは考えている。胚子や胎児が催奇性作用に対してもっとも感受性が高い期間を、奇形形成の臨界期という。心臓、中枢神経系、硬口蓋、外性器は、解剖学的に複雑に構成されている器官で、原則として長い奇形形成の臨界期を持つ。そのため、セシウム137が母親-胎児系に入り込むと、なによりもまず、解剖学的に複雑なこれらの器官が損傷を受ける（図1.9.1）。

　人びとの遺伝的欠陥の発生率が、主に放射能被曝の影響で年々上がっていることを考えると、母親-胎児系に入り込んだセシウム137の先天性奇形誘発因子としての重要性も増している。セシウム137は発育中の胎児の原基の栄養機能を障害し、直接的に胎児の細胞の代謝に悪影響を与え、胎盤の組織を障害する。奇形の形成にセシウム137が関与する可能性を考慮する必要がある。セシウム137の奇形形成に対する関与は、胎児の骨格骨の形成でとくに明瞭にみられる。放射性セシウムは骨原基の増殖過程の強度を低下させ、骨の低形成を引き起こす。セシウム137の蓄積が増すのに並行して、母親-胎児系では代謝過程が悪化する。セシウム137によって体内汚染されている状況では、胚子胎児発育の早期に形成される原基（上肢の骨原基）よりも、後の期間に形成される原基（下肢の骨原基）のほうがより強い悪影響を受ける。著者らは、白ラットとシリアンハムスターにオキシチアミンを投与して、B_1ビタミン欠乏症による代謝障害を母親-胎児系に起こす模擬実験を実施した。その実験結果でも、同様の効果が観察された[57]。

　セシウム137によって、先天性奇形以外に胚子と胎児の死亡が起きる可能性がある。

　母親の内分泌系がセシウム137によって悪影響を受けると、とくに子宮内発育の初期の段階で、卵巣ホルモンの産生が異常になる。

　その結果、胚の着床に対する子宮粘膜の受け入れ態勢が整わない事態が生じる。放射性物質が、卵子、受精卵-接合子、分割胚-桑実胚、胞胚に入り込むと、後になって発育中の胎児の組織に深刻な病変が生じる可能性がある。

　遺伝的な欠陥と内分泌状態の逆転の並存は、非常に頻繁にみられる。

図 1.9.1 ヒトの胚子胎児発育の臨界期の妊娠週（ムル・ミチ、1973）

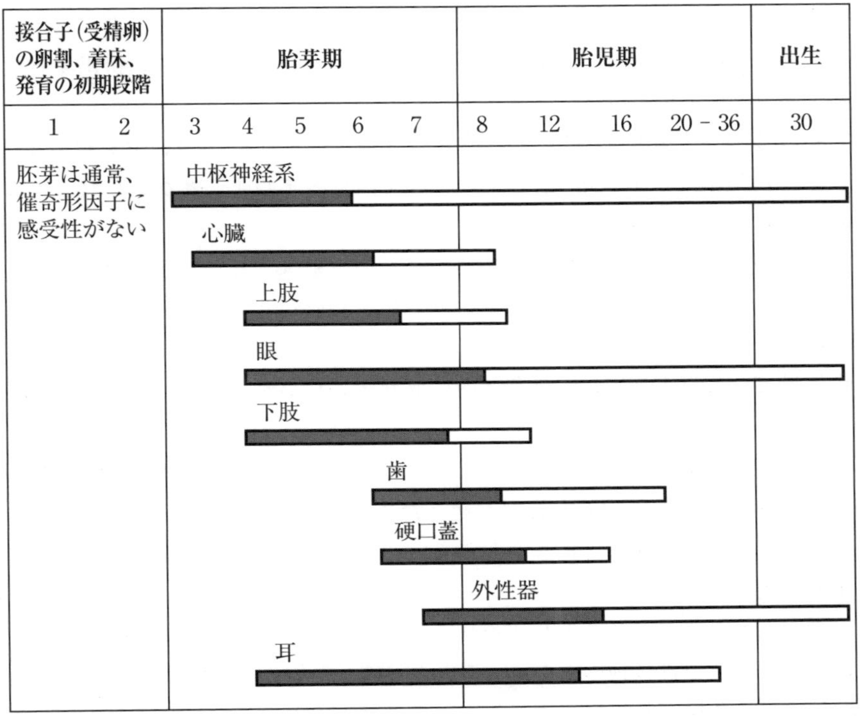

接合子(受精卵)の卵割、着床、発育の初期段階	胎芽期	胎児期	出生
1　　2	3　4　5　6　7	8　12　16　20－36	30

胚芽は通常、催奇形因子に感受性がない	中枢神経系
	心臓
	上肢
	眼
	下肢
	歯
	硬口蓋
	外性器
	耳

注：妊娠第2週までは催奇形因子の影響は通常、胚芽の死を招く。妊娠第3週から第8週までは大きな形態学的異常。妊娠第9週以降は原則として生理的な欠陥と小さな形態学的変異。

　　影つきの部分：催奇形因子にもっとも感受性が高い時期。

　　影なし部分：催奇形因子に対する胎児の感受性がそれよりも低い時期。

　すべての放射性物質、とくにセシウム137が体内に取り込まれると、その影響で子どもの親の世代の女性と男性の両方の生殖細胞のゲノムに欠陥が生じることは疑いようがない。しかし、化学的、生物学的な突然変異誘発物質の影響も無視するわけにはいかないこともたしかである。

　放射性セシウムが胎児期に、胎児の組織に影響する場合、粗大な奇形は生じないが、さまざまな臓器の細胞を障害する作用は持っている。セシウム137が胎児期に影響すると、セシウム137の病理作用は出生後の子どもに現れる可能性がある。胎児期や出生後の段階でセシウム137が作用すると、さまざまな臓器、とくに免疫系、内分泌系、神経系、心臓、肝臓、腎臓の高度

に分化した細胞が損傷を受ける。

　セシウム 137 は、主に母乳と人工栄養のための乳製品から哺乳期の乳児に入り込む。授乳期間中、母親は大量の放射性セシウムを母乳中に排出するため、母乳を子どもに与えることは容認できない。

　ベラルーシ共和国の RPL-99（放射能許容水準 − 99）では、セシウム 137 による汚染濃度が 100Bq/kg までの牛乳を消費にまわすことが許される。このため、PRL-99 に同意することは不可能である。

　成長中の子どもの体の細胞のエネルギー産生系は、とくこの細胞毒によって深刻な悪影響を受ける。内分泌機能と免疫機能が低下した状態で起きる病気は、たいていの場合、感染症である。その感染症によって、子どもの体を傷つけている真の病因、つまり体内に取り込まれた放射性セシウムの作用が覆い隠されてしまう。

　放射能汚染地域に住んでいたことがあるか、あるいは現在住んでいる両親に生まれた新生児に病的な経過が起きた場合、適切な診断を下すためには、子どもと母親の放射分析検査をおこない、体内の放射性セシウム濃度を測定する必要がある。

　病因論からみて診断を下し、それにもとづいて適切な治療を進めるためには、長寿命放射性核種のセシウム 137 が母親−胎児系に影響することによって起こる、胎児と新生児の放射能毒性症候群が実際に存在していることを受け入れる必要がある。診断や治療における誤りを避けるために、著者らは以前、この症候群を長寿命放射性核種の体内取り込み症候群の一変種として説明している[3]。

　年長の子どもの死亡例の臓器にもセシウム 137 の蓄積が認められた（図 1.9.2）。セシウム 137 は甲状腺、副腎、膵臓、心筋に高濃度で集積する特徴がある[49]。組織学的な検査でも、甲状腺、副腎、膵臓、心筋が障害されていた。胎児と新生児では、障害された重要臓器の細胞の変性と変性壊死は、たいていの病変部位で生命維持が不可能なほどであった。

　「免疫系の障害−感染症が進行する原因」。公式書類上には、子どもたちの死因はこう書かれている。しかし、セシウム 137 の影響による臓器の細胞障害に加えて、免疫系の障害もたしかに起きてくる。免疫系に障害があると、ありふれた細菌叢ですら身体に著しい悪影響を及ぼすだろう。そして結核、ウィルス性肝炎も人びとの集団で広く蔓延する。放射性セシウムによっ

図 1.9.2　大人と子どもの臓器のセシウム 137 濃度
　　　　　（1997 年に死亡したゴメリ州の住民）[6, 29]

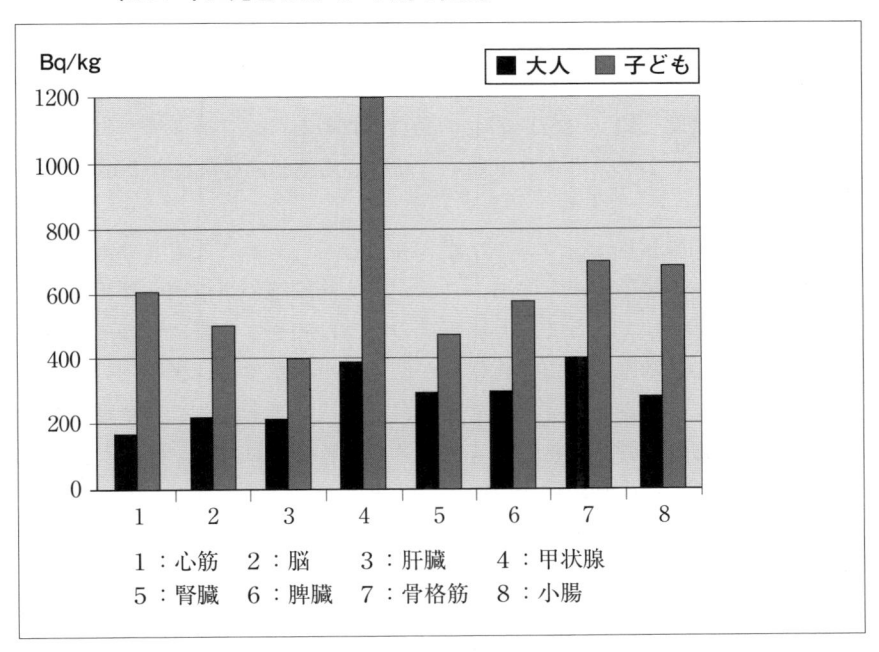

1：心筋　　2：脳　　3：肝臓　　4：甲状腺
5：腎臓　　6：脾臓　　7：骨格筋　　8：小腸

て肝実質細胞が障害される。それに加え免疫系、とくに、まず抑制性免疫が放射性セシウムで障害される。肝炎ウィルスが存在していると、抑制性免疫が低下することで、通常の方法では治療困難な慢性肝炎の急性増悪が起きる。中毒性の肝変性、肝硬変症、または肝臓の慢性変性による肝性脳症や肝不全が増え、一般的に広くみられるようになった。

　腎臓は放射性セシウムを体外に排泄する器官のひとつであり、腎臓で放射性セシウム濃度が高いことは偶然ではない（図 1.9.2）。

　腎臓のセシウム 137 濃度が高いと、大人だけでなく子どもでも糸球体装置と尿細管を障害する病理過程が進行する [5]。血管の病変が、糸球体に壊死性病変を引き起こし、腎不全の原因となっている。しかし、その腎臓血管病変の経過は、ほとんどの場合、潜伏性で症状が表に現れない。セシウム 137 の悪影響の結果、尿毒症になる。しかし、臨床医には尿毒症が突然発症したかのようにみえる。セシウム 137 の影響で、尿細管もひどく障害される。最近、ベラルーシでは腎臓に腫瘍性病変がある人びとの数が増えていることを述べ

ておかなければならない [30]。

　心臓は、機能するためにエネルギーを激しく消費する臓器の典型であり、セシウム 137 という毒物の影響で、もっとも早期に障害される臓器のひとつである。体内のセシウム 137 濃度 63.35 ± 3.58Bq/kg の実験動物では、体内セシウム 137 濃度 5.43 ± 0.87Bq/kg の動物と比較して、エネルギー回路の主要酵素であるクレアチンホスフォキナーゼの心筋細胞内の活性が 50％低下していた [47]。

　心筋細胞の細胞質にセシウム 137 が入り込むと、それにともない心筋細胞ではエネルギーの産生が不足する。これが、心筋細胞の蛋白同化作用が低下する主な原因となって、とくに心筋線維の収縮に関与する蛋白質の生合成を低下させる。心筋細胞の蛋白同化作用が低下した状況では、細胞内の修復再生過程が劇的に障害される。そうすると、身体的なストレス、神経精神医学的な影響、毒物の影響など、どのようなストレスを受けても、心臓と全心血管系の活動の深刻な異常が顕著な臨床症状をともなって起きてくる可能性がある。このような例が拡張型心筋症である。拡張型心筋症は、収縮能の喪失を伴う心臓壁の嚢状の拡張で 30 ～ 50 歳で発病する。拡張型心筋症の罹患率は年々上昇している。拡張型心筋症の増加は偶然ではない。チェルノブイリ原発事故から 24 年以上がたち、心血管系を含む重要臓器系が発達する重要な時期をチェルノブイリ原発事故後に過ごした子どもたちが成長したためである。

　心臓に対する放射性セシウムの有害作用の指標となるのは、心筋の収縮と弛緩を制御する心筋刺激伝導系の構造と機能の異常である。放射性セシウムは低濃度であっても、刺激伝導系を通る電気パルスの伝導障害を引き起こす可能性がある。この伝導障害はさまざまな心筋伝導ブロックの形をとって現れる。子どもの心筋活動の異常の頻度と、体内のセシウム 137 濃度とのあいだに相関関係があることが判明している [45, 46, 47]。

　子どもの心筋活動の異常も、遺伝子活動の調節を含む、ヒトと動物の体の調整過程の存在が理解できるようになった段階で説明可能になると著者らは考えている。細胞内遺伝装置の活動の調節（刺激）系の機能を阻害する外部環境要因は、多くの病気を引き起こす誘発因子となるであろう。遺伝的な欠陥がある場合、放射性セシウムは心血管系の細胞のエネルギー産生過程を阻害することによって生命維持に向けられている代償的適応過程を妨害し、病

理変化の発現を招く。

体内のセシウム 137 濃度が上昇するにつれ、心機能障害の発症率が上昇し、心臓病変もより重篤化する。セシウム 137 濃度が上昇すると、大量の心筋細胞が死滅する。大量の心筋細胞が死滅する結果起きるのは、上記の拡張型心筋症や突発する心停止である。

子どもの内分泌異常の原因となるものは子宮内の発育期間にある。子宮内の発育期間に放射性セシウムが影響して起きる胎児の副腎の低形成と、それに関連するホルモンの産生不全がそれである。胎児の発育期間と出生後の子どもの発育時に、セシウム 137 の毒作用による副腎の損傷とホルモンの産生不全がみられる。 副腎のホルモン産生不全は、コルチゾールの産生でもっとも明瞭になる。膵臓、生殖腺、そしてもちろん甲状腺についても同じことがいえる。甲状腺に対する損傷は、セシウム 137 に加えてヨウ素 131 も関係している。セシウム 137 とヨウ素 131 の 2 つの放射性核種は、ベラルーシのみならず、西ヨーロッパの人びとの健康にも恐るべき事態をもたらした。その結果は、甲状腺癌と自己免疫性甲状腺炎の高い罹患率である。甲状腺癌と自己免疫性甲状腺炎の発病には、ヨウ素 131 が主導的な役割を担っているという見方が確立されている。著者らが得た知見では、セシウム 137 も甲状腺の細胞に集中的に吸収される。そのため、セシウム 137 も、ヨウ素 131 に劣らぬ重要な役割を甲状腺癌と自己免疫性甲状腺炎の発病に担っていると考えられる。セシウム 137 は、甲状腺の細胞のエネルギー産生をむしばみ、細胞死をもたらすだけでなく、細胞の修復と細胞内の修復を障害し、細胞の分化も妨げる。さらに、細胞の構成成分が免疫系に対して抗原となることを促進する。加えて、セシウム 137 はリンパ球の細胞分画の均衡を乱して抑制性免疫を低下させ、免疫系に悪影響を与える。

自己抗体と免疫担当細胞が甲状腺を攻撃する免疫反応が起き、自己免疫性甲状腺炎を発病する。そして、自己免疫性甲状腺炎を背景に甲状腺癌が発生してくる。

甲状腺に対する放射性セシウムの影響は、甲状腺や甲状腺の組織の活動に対する免疫調節の異常という観点から考慮するだけでなく、甲状腺の細胞の構成要素に対する損傷の性質からも考慮する必要がある。

短寿命放射性核種のヨウ素 131 の崩壊は、エネルギー放出をともなって細胞内の遺伝装置の構造を破壊する。ヨウ素 131 の場合、前述の病理過程は比

較的急速に進行する。

　免疫系は、子宮内の発育期にセシウム137の影響にさらされる。子宮内でセシウム137の影響を受けると、子どもに免疫不全が起きてくることは、臨床的にも実験的にも確認されている。子どもの免疫不全が潜在性の状態にとどまっている場合には、アレルギー性疾患や感染症が高い頻度で発症してくる。セシウム137が免疫産生器官に大量に入り込むと、母親－胎児系の免疫的連関と免疫調節関係が障害される。加えて、出生前死亡や多因子性グループに属する先天性奇形などの子宮内発育異常が起きてくる。

　出生後の発育時に、セシウム137が子どもの免疫産生器官に入り込むと、慢性の免疫不全状態になる。この慢性免疫不全は、腫瘍性疾患と感染症が発病するひとつの原因となる。子どもたちにリンパ系組織と造血系組織の悪性新生物が増えていることについても述べておく必要がある[30]。

　神経系は放射性セシウムの影響で傷つけられる。それは子宮内発育の時期からはじまっている。一連の対立遺伝子の活性の欠如などの遺伝的な素因があると、セシウム137の影響でヒトと一連の実験動物に中枢神経系の奇形が起きる。その中枢神経系の奇形は多因子性グループに属している。外脳症、頭蓋脳ヘルニアのような奇形がもっとも頻繁にみられる。セシウム137の影響は、胎児の発育期に細胞内修復機能にたけた活発な神経細胞を傷つける。そして神経系に特有の構造を形成することを障害する。セシウム137が出生後の発育期に子どもの神経系の細胞に入り込んでも、まったく同じ作用が現れる。出生後にセシウム137が入り込むと、神経系の細胞では生理活性を持つ物質の代謝が徹底的に阻害される[31]。中枢神経系の悪性疾患がどんどん増加しているのは、放射性セシウムが中枢神経系の組織に大量に入り込むことが原因となっていると著者らは考えている。このことは統計データからも確認されている。1992年から2001年にかけて、脳腫瘍はリンパ系組織や造血系組織の悪性新生物とともに、ベラルーシの子どもたちの腫瘍性疾患の構成のなかで主要な位置を占めてきた[30]。

　以上のことから、セシウム137については以下のように考えるべきである。
　　1）体細胞の突然変異過程を引き起こす原因であり、悪性新生物増加の主要な原因のひとつである。
　　2）生殖細胞の突然変異過程の原因であり、次世代の出生前、出生後発育における病理変化の基盤になる。

3）重要臓器の細胞内エネルギー産生過程を阻害する要因であり、以下のことを招く。
- a）体内のセシウム137濃度が20〜30Bq/kgの比較的低濃度では、セシウム137の調節不全作用が体内の調節過程を混乱させる。セシウム137やその他の放射性物質は親世代の生殖細胞に対して突然変異誘発作用を持っており、潜在性の遺伝性素因を基盤とする病理過程や病気の発症に関与する。そのような例として、先天性奇形と子どもの不整脈がある。
- b）体内のセシウム濃度が50Bq/kg以上の高濃度では、放射性物質を取り込んだ細胞で細胞内のエネルギー産生装置の破壊をともなう変性壊死が進行する。この例は拡張型心筋症である。

チェルノブイリ原発事故の被災地で多くの病気の罹患率が上昇している。その根本的な原因はこの中にあるだろう。

第 **2** 部
チェルノブイリ原発事故で被災した ウクライナ住民の生殖に関する健康状態

2.1 放射能汚染郡の出生率の動向

　人類の科学技術史上最悪の大惨事、チェルノブイリ原発事故のあと、人びとの生殖機能を示す統計指標に否定的な傾向が現れ、ますます悪化している。そのため人びとの生殖機能は、多くの研究者の注目するところとなった[1, 2]。放射能汚染地域で暮らす人びとの出生率が低下した原因は、とくに緊急の究明を要する課題である。

　大量の人工放射性物質が破壊された原子炉から環境中に降下し、ウクライナの被災地域に放射能に関するさまざまな問題をもたらした。チェルノブイリの原発事故から1年後、セシウム137の土壌汚染が555kBq/m^{2}を超える郡は放射線厳重管理区域に指定され、住民に対する放射線防護措置が導入された。1987年に、キエフ州のポレスコエ郡とイワンコフ郡、ジトミール州のルギヌイ郡とナロジッチ郡、チェルニゴフ州のコゼレフ郡、レプキン郡、チェルニゴフ郡が放射線厳重管理区域に指定された。1988年、コゼレフ郡、レプキン郡、チェルニゴフ郡の3郡は放射線厳重管理区域から外されたが、ジトミール州のオブルチ郡が放射線厳重管理区域に指定された。その後の数年間に、放射線厳重管理区域は12の州の74郡まで増加した。最初の5郡の放射能汚染レベルは深刻なままだった。ウクライナの放射能汚染地域での居住に関する指定計画のすべてをこの5郡にみることができる。すなわち、避難区域、無条件（義務的）移住区域、補償自主移住区域、放射線厳重管理区域である[3]。これらの郡からは、1990～1992年のあいだに相当数の住民が移住すると予想されていた。

　チェルノブイリ原発事故直後の緊急期に、放射性ヨウ素によって、とくに子どもたちの甲状腺が汚染された[4]。放射線厳重管理区域の全郡で、平均被曝線量は緊急事態時の基準である30センチグレイ（cGy）を超えていた。さ

らに、ナロジッチ郡（52.6cGy）とポレスコエ郡（44.1cGy）では成人の被曝線量も緊急時の基準を超えていた。それらの郡に住む住民の1996〜2000年までの全身累積被曝線量を計算すると、1人あたり平均で6.0〜29.9mSvに達した。

　チェルノブイリ原発事故後の最初の4年間、放射線厳重管理区域に指定された郡にある175カ所の居住地の人びとの全身被曝線量は、年間1mSvを超えていた。これは、チェルノブイリ原発事故による放射能汚染度の高いウクライナが住民居住計画で決めた年間許容被曝線量を超えていた（1991年）。

　1986年にチェルノブイリ原発事故が起きるまでは、調査対象の郡の人口統計には、出生率が高く、子沢山で、転出率が低く、死亡率も低く、都市化が進み、人口密度も高いという特徴があった。人口統計の指標値は小さな変動を示したが、ウクライナ全州の平均値とほぼ同じだった。

　チェルノブイリ原発事故の後、人びとの生殖過程と居住状況は劇的に変化した。1986年の避難と1990年にはじまった住民の移住によって人口が減少した。人口の性別年齢構成もいびつになった。チェルノブイリ原発事故直後の2カ月間に、2市と69村の住民9万1600人が放射能で汚染された郡から避難させられた。放射能汚染地域からの組織化された移住の第二波は、政府の決定のもと1990年からはじまった。ウクライナ政府緊急事態省の公式データによれば、1986年から1995年までのあいだに112の居住地区が移住地区に指定され、約16万3000人が自主的に移住した。引き続く1996〜2000年の5年間で移住は大幅に減った。2000年以降は、散発的な移住になるまで減少した。

　2011年の初頭、無条件（義務的）移住区域（ゾーンⅡ）のジトミール州には、まだ532家族が残っている。しかも、そのうち113家族には、14歳以下の子どもがいる。そして居住が法的に禁止されている避難区域（ゾーンⅠ）にも、150人の「自責定住者」たちが住んでいる[7]。現在、放射能汚染地域の人びとの大部分は、補償自主移住区域（ゾーンⅢ）と放射線厳重管理区域（ゾーンⅣ）に住んでいる。

　強制移住と自発的な退去のため、放射能汚染郡では、生殖年齢にある女性たちの人口構成に占める割合が減り、2000年にはチェルノブイリ原発事故以前の3分の1になった。年齢層別にみると、20〜29歳の年齢層の女性の人口は約63％に減少した（図2.1.1）。出生数の3分の2は、この年齢層の女性

図 2.1.1 1981 年から 2000 年までのウクライナの放射能汚染郡と対照郡における
         20 歳から 29 歳の女性人口の変遷
         （1981 年から 1985 年までの指標の平均値を 100％とした）

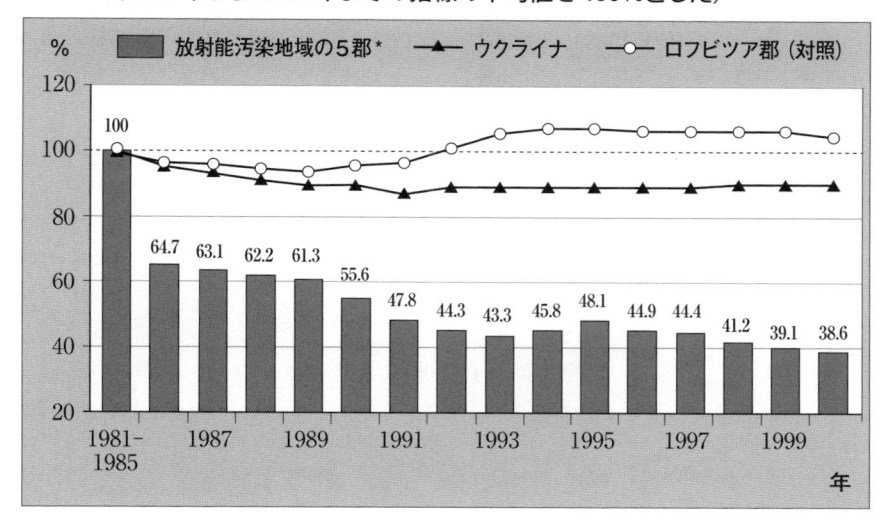

```
%        ■ 放射能汚染地域の5郡*   ▲ ウクライナ   ○ ロフビツア郡（対照）
120
100  100
           64.7  63.1  62.2  61.3
 80                             55.6
                                     47.8  44.3  43.3  45.8  48.1  44.9  44.4
 60                                                                         41.2  39.1  38.6
 40
 20
   1981-    1987    1989    1991    1993    1995    1997    1999
   1985                                                              年
```

＊：郡構成の中にイワンコフ、ポレスコエ、ルギヌイ、ナロジッチ、オブルチの各郡が含まれる。

たちによってもたらされる。一方、対照郡では、20 ～ 29 歳の年齢層の女性数は増加傾向を示した。平均年齢は 2.5 歳上昇し、人口減少過程の激化を示した。

　ウクライナの自然人口動態分析では、1986 ～ 2000 年にかけて、チェルノブイリ原発事故以前に比べて出生率が大きく低下した。このことは、粗出生率 ［訳注：粗出生率とは人口 1000 人あたりのその年の出生数］ に否定的な影響を与えた（表 2.1.1）。

　放射能汚染郡の当初の出生率（1981 ～ 1985 年）は 14.1‰だった。チェルノブイリ原発事故後の 5 年間で、出生率は 13.7‰（1986 年）から 8.8‰（2000 年）に低下した。これは当初の値の 63％である。チェルノブイリ原発事故後 2 年目の 1987 年に、30％にもなる出生率のもっとも顕著な低下がみられた（図 2.1.2）。出生率がこの時期に急激に低下した原因は、住民、とくに都市部の住民が妊娠出産を控えたためである。これは、チェルノブイリ原発事故に対するストレス反応として起きた。

　1981 ～ 1985 年までの値との比較で、出生率の最低値は 2000 年に記録された。放射能汚染地域と非汚染地域の両方で、出生率は 1991 年以降、最高水準

表 2.1.1 放射能汚染地域と対照地域における 1981 〜 2000 年の粗出生率の変遷

地域	出生率 (‰)			1981 〜 1985 年と比較しての変化率 (%)	
	1981-1985	1986-1990	1991-2000	1986-1990	1991-2000
ルギヌイ郡	15.0	13.8	12.7	-8.0	-15.0
ナロジッチ郡	11.7	11.0	14.4	-6.0	+23.0
オブルチ郡	13.8	12.2	10.7	-12.0	-23.0
イワンコフ郡	12.5	10.8	9.1	-14.0	-27.0
ポレスコエ郡	15.9	13.5	12.1	-15.0	-24.0
放射能汚染地域の5郡	14.1	12.9	10.9	-9.0	-23.0
ロフビツア郡 (対照)	12.2	11.9	9.0	-3.0	-26.0
ウクライナ	15.2	14.2	9.6	-7.0	-37.0

出典：ウクライナ国家統計委員会のデータに基づき著者が計算した。

図 2.1.2 1981 〜 1994 年までの放射能汚染されたイワンコフ郡と、汚染されていないロフビツア郡の粗出生率の変遷
（1981 年の値を 100% とした）

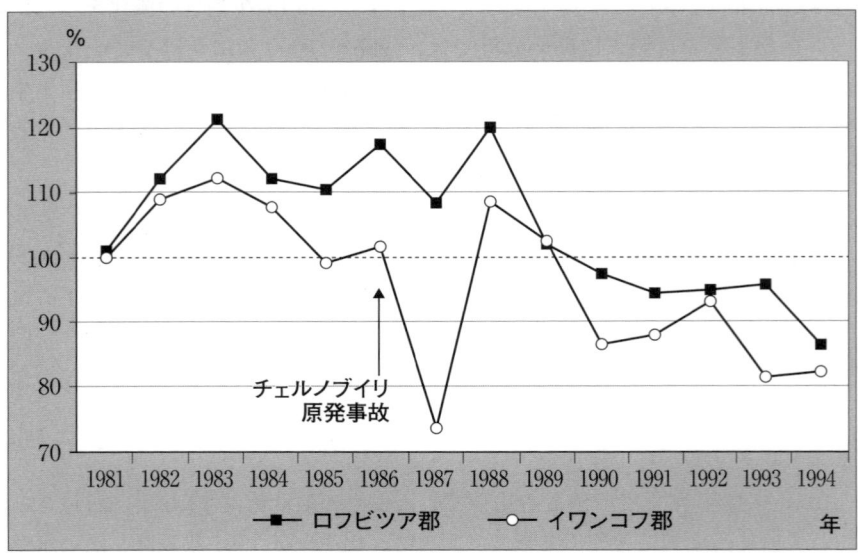

図 2.1.3 1986 年から 2007 年までのウクライナ住民の
　　　　粗出生率の変遷と社会経済的変容

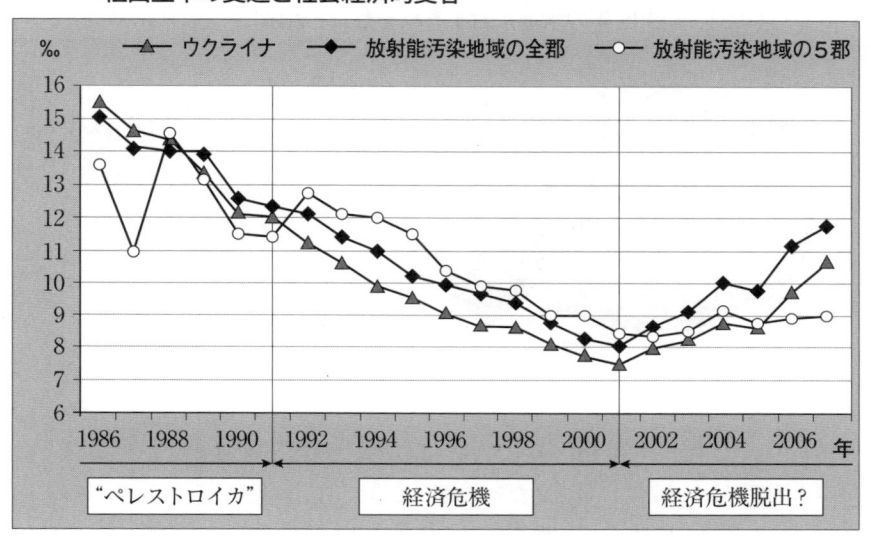

から低下した。これは 1990 〜 1991 年に起きた社会体制と生活経済の崩壊過程と、その後の更なる経済悪化が背景にある（図 2.1.3）。

　人口調査の対象となる住民の年齢構成の変化が、粗出生率の変遷に影響する。とくに、15 〜 49 歳の生殖年齢にある女性が全人口に占める割合の変化と、生殖年齢の女性集団をさらに細分化した各年齢群が占める相対的な割合に影響される。

　1986 〜 2000 年にかけて、放射能汚染地域では、15 〜 19 歳の最若年層の女性を除くほとんどの年齢層の女性で出生率が減少した。チェルノブイリ原発事故後の 2 年目に、45 〜 49 歳の高齢層の女性群と、15 〜 19 歳の最若年層の女性群では出生率が増加した。しかし、この 2 つの群が粗出生率に寄与するところは少ないので、粗出生率の変化にはほとんど影響がなかった。放射能汚染郡では、全調査期間を通じて出生率が低下した。非汚染郡でも、1991 年から出生率が低下しはじめた。これは、20 〜 34 歳の年齢層の女性の出生活動が 80％以上も低下したことが原因である。放射能汚染地域では、新生児全体に第一子が占める割合が圧倒的に多かった。

　放射能汚染郡の出生活動の急速な減少は、合計特殊出生率［訳注：合計特殊出

第 2 部　55

図 2.1.4　1986～2000 年にかけての放射能汚染郡の出生率低下に対する個別の人口統計学的要因の寄与率（1981～1985 年の水準に対するパーセント表示）

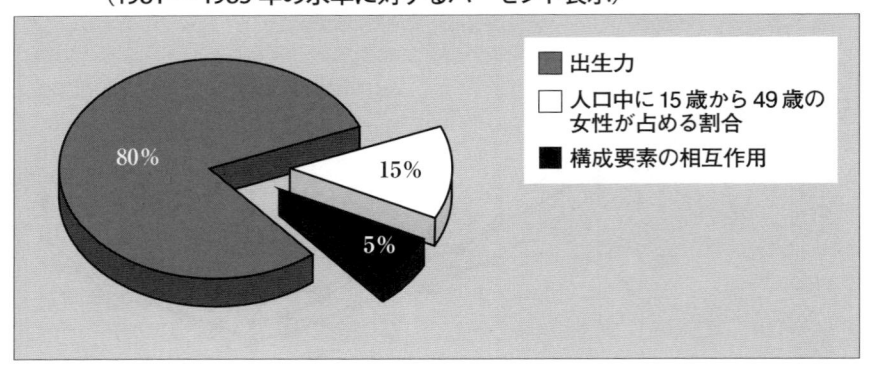

凡例：
- 出生力
- 人口中に 15 歳から 49 歳の女性が占める割合
- 構成要素の相互作用

80%　15%　5%

生率は、1 人の女性が一生のうちで産む子どもの平均人数〕の低下も意味している。合計特殊出生率は 1986 年には 2.2 だったが、2001 年には 1.2 に低下した。都市部では 1.8 から 1.1 に低下し、地方では 2.3 から 1.4 に低下した。1991～2002 年にかけて、81～84％を占める新生児の大部分が、30 歳以下の女性に生まれた。つまり、放射能汚染地域のみならず、ウクライナ全体でも、女性の出生活動は比較的早い年齢で切り上げられた。

2000 年には、放射能汚染地域の出生率は、人口の破局過程の起きる限界を越えて低下してしまった。その結果、放射能汚染郡では、人口統計的にも、社会的にも、発展に必須とされる前提条件が失われた。この破局的な出生率の低下は、チェルノブイリ原発事故後に起きた生態学的、社会経済学的変化に対して人びとが順応したことの現れであると学者たちは考えている。

成分分析の結果では、1986～2000 年までの放射能汚染郡における出生率の低下に、出生力という因子が寄与した割合は 80％だった。他方、人口構成因子の寄与率は 15％だった。これらの 2 つの因子の影響が重なりあったことによる寄与率は 5％だった（図 2.1.4）。

ウクライナの世論調査の結果では、現在、人びとが子どもをつくろうとしない理由の第 1 位は、多くの家庭がおかれている厳しい経済状態である。ウクライナの女性回答者の 43％が、望みどおりの数の子どもを産むのに必要な条件として、所得水準の上昇を挙げていた[8]。望みどおりの数の子どもを持つか否かを夫婦が決定する上で、住宅状況（17.9％）と家族に子どもを保育

表 2.1.2　1986 年から 2007 年までの、ウクライナと放射能汚染郡人口集団の出生率の主な指標

年	人口 1000 人当たりの出生数			女性 1 人に当たりの平均出生数		
	ウクライナ	放射能汚染群 RCD*	ウクライナに対する%	ウクライナ	放射能汚染群 RCD*	ウクライナに対する%
1986-1990	14.1	13.4	95.0	2.2	2.1	95.5
1991-1995	10.8	11.1	102.8	1.6	1.7	106.2
1996-2000	8.4	9.0	107.2	1.2	1.4	108.3
2001	7.7	8.2	106.5	1.1	1.3	118.2
2002	8.1	8.7	107.4	1.1	1.3	118.2
2003	8.5	9.2	108.2	1.2	1.4	116.7
2004	9.0	9.8	108.9	1.2	1.4	116.7
2005	9.0	9.6	106.7	1.2	1.4	116.7
2006	9.8	10.5	107.2	1.3	1.5	115.4
2007	10.2	11.0	107.9	1.3	1.5	115.4

＊：チェルノブイリ原発事故で被災したウクライナの郡のすべて
出典：ウクライナ国家統計委員会のデータに基づき著者が計算した。

する時間がないこと（10.6％）も大きな影響を与えていた。

　ウクライナ国立科学アカデミー社会学研究所がおこなった社会学的調査によれば、ゾーンⅡに住む回答者の 10 分の 1 と、ゾーンⅢの回答者の 6 分の 1 が、将来子どもを持つつもりがない理由として、チェルノブイリ原発事故の余波を挙げていた。反対に"汚染されていない"郡の住民は、この要素を考慮に入れていなかった[9]。加えて、放射能汚染地域住民の回答者は子どもを持たない理由として、何にもまして経済的な要因を挙げた。　放射能汚染された郡では出生率が長く低下し続けた後、2002 年から出生率が徐々に上昇しはじめた（表 2.1.2）。

　2002 ～ 2007 年にかけて、粗出生率は 34.1％増加した（都市部で 34.7％、地方では 33.5％の上昇）。最近 6 年間、放射能汚染郡の女性の出生活動が全ての年齢層で上昇している。とくに 25 ～ 39 歳の女性では毎年 10％ずつ上昇している。この年齢層は、第二子か第三子を産む時期である。

　都市部の 30 ～ 39 歳の女性で出生率がもっとも高くなった。これは以前に妊娠出産を先送りしたが、後でそれを埋め合わせるための妊娠出産をしたことと関係している。第一子と第二子を出産する年齢が多くの女性で高齢化

したという証拠がある。これに関連して、2002～2007年のあいだに第一子の出産年齢は、20～24歳の年齢層から25～29歳の年齢層へとずれた。第二子の出産年齢は、25～29歳の年齢層から30～34歳の年齢層に移動した。第三子の出産年齢は、30～34歳の年齢層から35～39歳の年齢層に移動した。出産年齢の高齢化は出生順位別の出生数の構成の変化を示している。

チェルノブイリ原発事故の余波のため、多くの女性が妊娠することを控え、子どもを持つことを先送りした。しかし後に、この埋め合わせをする出産の増加が起きた。この出産増加は、2つの正反対の理由で起きた。ひとつは住民への福祉がいくらか改善したことであり、もうひとつは、新たな生活状況に社会が徐々に順応したことである。それに加え、人口政策に基づく出産奨励策が実施されたことも出産増加の原因になった（出産時に限られるが、2005年4月1日から、一定の効果を期待できる手厚い援助がなされるようになった）。

特殊な刺激要因が出生率を押し上げた面もある。1983～1986年に生まれた女性が生殖年齢に入ったことで、出産する年齢層の女性の割合が一時的に増えたことである。放射能汚染郡の人びとの年齢層別出生活動を居住地別に分析した。すると、都市部と農村部の女性では年齢層別の出生率に違いがあることがわかった。

農村部の女性では、24歳以下の年齢層の出生活動がはっきりと大幅に増大していた。放射能汚染郡の農村地帯では、20歳以下の女性の出生活動が都市部の2倍で、20～24歳の年齢層の女性の出生活動は、都市部より1.5倍高かった。

つまり、放射能汚染地域の農村地帯の女性の過半数（60％）は、25歳以下の年齢で出生活動をしていた。都市部の30～39歳の年齢層の女性は、農村部の同年齢層の女性より第二子と第三子の出生数の合計で勝っていた。しかし、これはむしろ、都市部の女性が第一子を産むのをしばしば先送りするため、第二子と第三子の出産年齢が高くなる一方で、農村部では伝統的に若くして結婚し、若いうちに子どもをつくる傾向があることを意味している。都市部の女性は当初低い出生率を示していた。しかし、2002年以降、とくに34～44歳の年齢層の女性が積極的に出生活動にたずさわるようになってきた。

この10年間に起きた放射能汚染郡の出生率の変動にともない、この地域の女性の年齢別の出生活動様式が大きく変化した。いまの若い人びとは、20年

前よりも高齢になってから出生活動をはじめる。現在の出生水準のかなりの部分は若い女性たちだけでなく、25歳以上の社会的により成熟した女性たちによっても担われている。

　チェルノブイリ原発事故後、放射能汚染郡では女性の年齢層による出生率に変化が生じた。そのおおまかな傾向を、女性の分娩時の平均年齢を指標として追跡することができる。分娩時の女性の平均年齢はチェルノブイリ原発事故の後、12年間は事実上変化しなかった（1986年は24.1歳で、1998年は23.8歳だった）。しかし、1998〜2007年にかけて分娩時の女性の平均年齢は急速かつ着実に上がっていった。この間に、女性の分娩時の平均年齢は1.7歳上昇し、2007年には25.5歳になった。

　ウクライナでは、2005年以降、州の人口政策で幼い子どものいる家庭に対する物質的な援助が強化された。子どもの誕生時の一時的な援助は、ヨーロッパでも最高の水準にまで劇的に引き上げられた。この援助は2008年にさらに強化された。しかし、政府の実施する政策に対する世論調査から、子どもの誕生時の一時的な手厚い援助は、大部分（87.4％）の回答者にとって、子どもをつくるか否かという判断にまったく影響を与えていないことが明らかになった[10]。出産時に一時的な支援をしても、出生率に対しては持続的な影響力はない。これは低出生率の問題を早急に解決しようとしてきた多くの国々が経験したことで、すでに確認済みである。さらに今後の10年間で、出生活動がもっとも盛んな年齢層にある女性の割合が減ると専門家たちは予想している。この人口構成の変化が出生率に与える影響は非常に大きい。そのため、ウクライナは新たな困難に直面することになる。

　このように、チェルノブイリ原発事故以降、ウクライナの放射能汚染郡に住む女性の出生率様式は、人口を維持してゆくことにおいて脅威となる性質を持っている。現在の出生率の指標のいくつかは、ウクライナ全体の状況を考えればいくらか「高い」といえるが、国際的な人口統計の基礎的指標からすれば極端に低い。2002年からみられる出生率の上昇傾向は、それまで妊娠して子どもをつくることを先送りしてきた25〜39歳の女性が、それを埋め合わせるために出生活動を高めはじめたことに起因する。また、1983〜1986年に生まれた女性が出産年齢に入り、一時的に出生活動をする女性集団が補充されたこと、2005年から人口政策措置が実施されたことも、放射能汚染郡とウクライナ全体で出生率の上昇をうながした主な要因となっている。

2.2 人びとの生殖損失の特性評価と出生率の変遷への関与

チェルノブイリ原発事故直後の緊急事態以降の期間に、放射能汚染地域の人びとの出生率低下を招いた主な要因は、生まれた子どもの数にあった。出生率が低いと、生殖損失*がその社会の人口再生産に悪影響を与える。

> *生殖損失：この指標は望まれた妊娠100例あたりの、自然流産数、医療上の必要性による人工妊娠中絶数、死産数と生後6日以内の子どもの死亡数の合計。

チェルノブイリ原発事故の後、放射能汚染郡では生殖損失率が絶え間なく上昇した。生殖損失が粗出生率の低下に寄与する割合は1987年には3.5％以下だった。しかし、1994年には、郡によって異なるものの、9.4～25.0％の範囲におよんだ。生殖損失率が出生率に与える否定的影響はナロジッチ郡（25.0％）、ポレスコエ郡（18.6％）、イワンコフ郡（15.5％）で非常に大きかった。放射能"非汚染"地域では、出生水準が生殖損失によって平均1.1％低下した。

それぞれの郡における生殖損失の量的特徴が示すところでは、すでに1986～1990年の期間において、ルギヌイ郡とポレスコエ郡では、生殖損失の顕著な過剰が起きていた（対照と比べてルギヌイ郡では5.3倍、ポレスコエ郡では8.1倍になっていた）（表2.2.1）。ジトミール州のナロジッチ郡をのぞく全調査対象郡で、1991年から生殖損失率が上昇し、否定的な傾向がみられる[11]。

生殖損失の構成のうち、85％以上が自然流産であった。自然流産のウクライナ総人口における頻度は、いろいろな報告によれば、5～25％の範囲に及んでいる[12, 13]。しかし、早期の流産は全妊娠例の8％で起きているのだが、多くの場合、妊婦本人にも気づかれていない[14]。政府の統計資料によれば、1986～1999年にかけて調査対象郡で記録された早期流産の平均発症率は、全妊娠の3.5～5.6％の範囲内にあった。公式には世界で記録された上限を超えていない[15]。

1983～1985年に比べ、2000年には生殖損失率は調査対象郡で2.4倍に増加した。一方、非汚染地域では、1.5倍の増加にとどまった。放射能汚染郡における生殖損失率の上昇は、統計的にも有意であった（$p<0.05$）。生殖損失率の年平均上昇率は、分析対象郡の平均で、希望妊娠100例に対し0.27例であった。1991～1992年に生殖損失率の最高値が記録された。それはチェルノブイリ事故前の水準の2.5倍以上であった[16]。

表 2.2.1 チェルノブイリ原発事故前後の放射能汚染郡と"非汚染"郡における生殖損失の量的特性評価(望まれた妊娠 100 例に対するパーセント表示)

郡	生殖損失			1983-1985 年に対する比		1983-1985 と比較した生殖損失の過剰	
	1983-1985	1986-1990	1991-1999	1986-1990	1991-1999	1986-1990	1991-1999
ルギヌイ	3.54	5.93	5.99	1.68	1.69	+2.39	+2.45
ナロジッチ	6.29	4.98	4.76	0.79	0.76	−1.31	−1.53
オブルチ	1.67	2.54	5.52	1.52	3.31	+0.87	+3.85
イワンコフ	4.32	5.33	9.73	1.23	2.25	+1.01	+5.41
ポレスコエ	3.87	7.50	8.26	1.94	2.13	+3.63	+4.39
放射能汚染地域の5郡	2.68	4.21	6.94	1.57	2.59	+1.53	+4.26
ロフビツア	4.10	4.55	7.76	1.11	1.89	+0.45	+3.66

　自然流産と早期新生児期の幼児死亡による生殖損失の相対危険率の増大が、1986 年から調査地域で記録され、統計学的にも有意差を認めた ($p<0.05$)。生殖損失の相対危険率の増大は、放射能汚染郡の住民の放射線被曝の合計集団実効線量と相関していた[17]。

　放射能汚染された居住地に住み、全身放射線被曝の総累積線量がかなり高い女性では、放射能非汚染地域の女性と比べ、自然流産が起きる危険性が高いことが確認されている[18]。

　生殖損失率の上昇は、妊婦の健康状態の悪化を背景にして起きた。放射能汚染郡では、1987 年以降、後期妊娠中毒症(1.5 〜 2.3 倍)と妊娠性貧血(10.0 〜 13.8 倍)の発病率が年々上昇する傾向がみられた。その結果、分娩時合併症の発病率も上昇した。放射能汚染郡では、不幸な結果に終わる妊娠の発生率はほぼ 2.1 倍に増加した。その原因は自然流産である。放射能汚染郡では、1986 年以降、妊娠第 22 〜 27 週で自然流産してしまうことが多くなっている。1989 〜 1990 年に、妊娠第 22 〜 27 週の自然流産が全自然流産に占めた割合は、放射能汚染郡で 19％だったのに対し、放射能非汚染郡では 10％だった[11]。自然流産の主な原因のひとつは先天性奇形であり、それは生殖損失の主な原因のひとつでもある。

　ウクライナとベラルーシの科学者たちの研究によって、先天性異常、発育欠陥、生殖損失の数が増加したことが示された。しかし、原子放射線の影響に関する国連科学委員会(UNSCEAR)は、2000 年、チェルノブイリ原

発事故による放射性物質の影響が原因で先天性障害が増えたとはいえないと結論した。この結論は、電離放射線の線量依存効果に関する世界の放射線生物学の知識に基づいてなされた。しかし、ウクライナ政府の被曝線量の評価方法には一貫性がない。またチェルノブイリ原発事故直後の1986年の推定被曝線量には誤りがある。そのため、ウクライナ国民の公式放射線被曝線量は著しく過小評価されていることに注意する必要がある[19]。ウクライナ政府は、世界中で実施されている放射能汚染事故時の体系的な分析法によって推定被曝線量を計算したわけではない。ウクライナ政府は、科学的に正当な根拠もなく、単純に低い線量係数（$9.4\mu Sv/Bq\cdot m^2$）を用いて、チェルノブイリ原発事故直後の1986年にウクライナ国民が全体として受けた緊急時被曝線量を計算した。このことは、チェルノブイリ原発事故の余波を小さく見せかけるためにおこなわれた。チェルノブイリ原発事故のあった1986年のウクライナ国民の放射線被曝線量は、1人の人が一生のあいだに受ける総被曝線量のわずか2～3％にすぎないというのが、ウクライナ政府の評価だった。一方、ソ連政府では90％を被曝したと評価した。もっとも控えめな推定でも、ウクライナの人びとは、確立された生涯許容被曝線量である7レムを超え、実際には最低10レムの放射線をすでに被曝してしまったか、今後被曝するだろう。放射線リスクの理論によれば、10レムの放射線量を被曝した場合、1000人中1人か、あるいは1000人の子孫のうちの1人が病気になる[19]。

　明らかになった変化から判断すると、放射能汚染地域に長く住むことは、生殖損失率を上昇させ、出生率を低下させる危険因子だといえる。しかし、現存する放射線被曝が、胎児の発育に与える影響を正確に見積もるには、個人ごとの被曝量に関するデータが必要である。残念なことに現在ウクライナには、このようなデータは存在していない。

　放射線被曝以外の要因も、生殖損失率に影響する。それらは具体的には、将来の親となる人びとの生殖健康の悪化、母親の年齢、生殖損失の症例の不完全な登録などである。

　放射能汚染地域の人びとの出生率の変化は、チェルノブイリ原発事故の影響と直接的なつながりがあり、人びとの繁殖を脅かす性質を持つようになっているということを分析結果は示している。出生率の指標、合計特殊出生率、生殖損失率は、調査対象となった人びとの周囲を取り巻く悪環境への適応力が衰えてきていることを示唆している。出生率に関する状況を改善するため

には政府レベルの決定が必要である。

　放射能汚染地域の出生率を上げるもっとも現実的な方法は、
　　1）放射線防護のために必要とされる措置を実施すること。
　　2）母親と子どもの健康を守ることに役立つ措置を実施すること。
　　3）正常な妊娠経過と正常な胎児の発育がみられる場合は、すべての希望される妊娠を維持すること。
　　4）人びとの生殖健康を強化するための措置を実施すること。

むすび

　このような小さな本で、チェルノブイリ原発事故の結果として起きた、放射能汚染地域のヒトの生殖の問題を書き尽くすことができないのは疑いない。しかし、人びとの高い死亡率と低い出生率が原因となって、人口動態が破局的な状況になっていることを認識する必要があるのは明らかである。出生率が低くなったのはかなりの程度、胎児の発育初期段階での死亡率が高くなったことに起因する。この事態を招いたさまざまな作用を挙げることができる。その主な原因のひとつは、現実に存在している放射線が人体に与える危険性を無視したことにある。その結果、人びとに効果的な防護措置が、まず国政レベルで十分に実施されなかった。

　科学的研究結果に基づいて結論すると、セシウム137が周辺の環境中に常に存在すると、当然人の体内にも存在するようになり、これが重要臓器の細胞にエネルギー欠乏を引き起こし、死に至る深刻な病理過程の進展を招く。

　とくに放射線は、中枢神経系や、内分泌器官を含む生殖系のすべての臓器に影響を与え、男性や女性の不妊症の原因のひとつになる。

　放射性物質の崩壊は両親の生殖細胞に突然変異を起こし、子孫、とくに胎児に、死亡や先天性奇形など、多くの場合、生命維持が不可能なほどの否定的な症状が現れる。

　母親−胎児系もまた、放射能の影響に非常に敏感である。母親−胎児系に入り込んだセシウム137は、子宮内での胎児死亡や先天性奇形の発症を助長する。ただし、ヒトの胎児の発育の初期段階で起きる病理過程を記録することはかなり困難である。そのため、医学的、遺伝学的、病理形態学的研究を組織し、胎児の発育病理に詳しい専門家に加わってもらう必要がある。この種の研究に必要不可欠なのは、胎児の身体とそれぞれの臓器、それに胎盤の放射性物質の濃度を測定することである。

　放射線の作用による胎児の発育障害は、子宮内での発育期間だけでなく、出生後の発育段階で症状として発現する可能性もある。重要なのは、子ども、

若者、および大人の病気の原因病理論的な診断を下すうえで、この基本原則を理解しておくことである。

大変残念なことに、体内に取り込まれた放射性物質がヒトの胎児の子宮内の発育過程にどのような影響をおよぼすのか、いまだにほとんど研究されていない。このため、大人を含む、出生前と出生後の発育過程で起きてくる病気を予防するための効果的な手段を開発して実施することが十分にできていない。

実際には、数多くの外部環境要因が発育中の身体に複合的な影響を与えていることに注目すべきである。生殖過程に否定的な影響を与える要因として、ニコチンやアルコール、それに麻薬が挙げられる。残念なことに、これらは放射能汚染郡の人びとに蔓延し、近年、身体に対する病原性作用を強めていることは疑いない。これらの要因によって、胎児期も含む高い罹病率と高い死亡率の主な原因である放射線の影響が、ある程度覆いかくされ、無視されている。

このため、放射線防護策以外にも、あらゆる手段を尽くして、放射能汚染地域の人びとのアルコール消費量を減らし、喫煙者の減少をうながす必要があることを強調しておく。

旧ソ連の崩壊によって深刻な社会経済的問題が発生し、それが直接の引き金となって医療問題も発生した。チェルノブイリ原発事故は社会経済的な危機を招き、状況をさらに悪化させた。

今日、放射線の影響にさらされている人びとの生存と将来の発展について、楽観的な見方をすることは困難である。医師の義務は、私たちが人びとの生命のために全力を尽くすことを命じている。私たちは、死の脅威にさらされている人びとを残して立ち去る権利を持っていない。

Yu. I. Bandazhevsky, N. F. Dubovaya

CONSEQUENCE OF THE CHERNOBYL DISASTER

REPRODUCTION OF HUMAN BEING IN CONDITION OF RADIATION EXPOSURE

The book is devoted to the processes of human reproduction in prolonged exposure of radionuclides. This book represents materials from long-term clinical and pathological observations, including experimental studies on laboratory animals, the effects of incorporated radionuclide Cs-137 on the female and male reproductive system, course of pregnancy and fetal development. Analyses of the results of epidemiological investigations of fertility and reproductive losses of the population living in territories of Ukraine affected by the Chernobyl nuclear power plant's accident.

The published materials can be of interest from a viewpoint of assessment of the impact of the real effect of radiation agents on reproductive health of inhabitants, in order to develop effective solutions to the current demographic problems.

Coordinating and Analytical Center «Ecology and Health», Kyiv– 2011

© Yu. I. Bandazhevsky, 2011
© N. F. Dubovaya, 2011

Preface of the authors

This book is devoted to the medical consequences of the Chernobyl disaster in 1986. The authors jointly have made their efforts toward comprehensive specifications of problems of human reproduction in the territories contaminated with radioactive agents.

The problem of human reproduction is one of the main problems of mankind. It is particularly urgent in countries most affected by the Chernobyl nuclear power plant disaster.

The demographic situation in Belarus, Ukraine, and Russian Federation is now catastrophic. Over the past 20 years, there have been observed a sharp decrease in the number of inhabitants in these countries, where its main reasons are the high mortality and low fertility rates. There are attempts to explain this phenomenon in relation with widespread negative public phenomena, such as smoking and alcoholism, as well as the low standard of living of the population.

However, these attempts do not take the effect of the radiation factor into account, having a huge power of influence on all the living on Earth. Population of the European part of the former Soviet Union confronted radiation agents in the 60s of the last century [1], having been in contact with them for 50 years, including the effect of radioactive nuclides of Chernobyl origin. The most widespread radiation agent in the environment is radio-cesium (Cs-137), which enters into the human organism with foodstuffs.

The authors wish to draw attention of the medical and scientific community to the existing demographic problem, from the standpoint of radiation impact factor in the human population.

The first section of this book presents materials from clinical and pathological observations, laboratory analysis, and experimental investigations of laboratory animals, characterizing the state of female and male reproductive systems, and the processes of intrauterine development of the embryo under the effects of radio-cesium incorporated into the organism.

The second section exhibits the results of epidemiological studies of fertility rate and reproductive losses of the inhabitants living in Ukraine suffering from the Chernobyl nuclear power plant disaster.

The authors hope that the materials in this publication will raise the interest of readers, especially medical professionals and scientists, involved in the impact of environmental factors on the human organism, and that they will also be taken into account for the development of measures aimed at the protection of health of the inhabitants living in the territories contaminated with radioactive elements.

Section 1

Incorporated radionuclide Cs-137 and the processes of human reproduction.

Chapter 1.1. § Radiological and demographic situation in the Republic of Belarus before and after the Chernobyl disaster.

One of the most actual issues which society faces any time, is the problem of the continuation of life for the future generations, in other words, production of the offspring carrying the best qualities of their ancestors.

For the last decade, in the territory of the Republic of Belarus, this problem does not find any proper solution. The birth rate sharply decreased, and mortality and morbidity of children after birth increased, as well as the number of children with abnormalities and congenital malformations. Naturally arises one question – What is it related with? Because of the deterioration of lives of people, including foodstuffs and medical care for mothers before and during pregnancy period? Or because of the influence of the huge number of factors of man-made origin to the human population?

If you deal with the problem of deterioration of the living standards of inhabitants in the recent years and its influence on the processes of reproduction, we can refer to the past and make sure that the hardest of deprivation of mankind (war, epidemics) could not lead to what we have today – in the Republic of Belarus – that mortality in the recent years exceeds the birth rate by 1.6 times.

The 20th century has brought up many sufferings and problems to the mankind. The development of nuclear technology has led to the fact that, starting from the 50s of the last century, the environment of human-biosphere is intensively filled with the new radioactive elements which formerly didn't exist on the Earth.

They include Cs-137, a long-lived radionuclide with a half-life period of 30 years. They enter the biosphere from radioactive waste, or from the products of nuclear explosions [40].

The sources of radioactive wastes are the nuclear reactors and the enterprises which are involved in the reprocessing of irradiated fuel. In the gaseous waste of reactors, Cs-137 is produced mainly from Xe-137, and then enters into the environment as liquid waste.

However, the most intensive environmental pollution of Cs-137 onto the living environment of the human being occurs in case of nuclear explosions, otherwise in case of accidents at the nuclear power plants, and such was the accident at the Chernobyl nuclear power plant in 1986.

Tremendous stream produced by thermal energy entrain the products of nuclear reaction into the stratosphere, where the products carry over long distances under the influence of air currents, causing global fallout (tropospheric and stratospheric) wherever on the surface of the Earth, regardless of the place where the explosion occurred.

The very physical nature of Cs-137 is a beta emitter, while Ba-137, which is a child product of Cs-137 with a half-life period of 2.55 minutes, emits gamma ray.

Cs-137 has been registered in the European part of USSR, including Belarus, since 1963. Based on the available research materials, the determination of this radionuclide in the foodstuff for mankind and animals can approve that the year of maximum fallout of radioactive nuclides in the Republic of Belarus before the Chernobyl catastrophe was exactly 1963[40].

The main food products forming a high level of Cs-137 in the organisms of inhabitants of Belarus in this period include milk, dairy products, bread, and meat of cattle and pigs. In particular, the concentration of Cs-137 in beef determined in results of research carried out by the Institute of Biophysics of the Ministry of Health care of USSR in the territory of Belorussian Polesie during the years of 1967-1970 was 700-8300 pCi/kg, and the content of Cs-137 in the daily diet ration of the inhabitants of several villages in the Gomel province, was 2059 pCi on average [40].

Thus, the inhabitants of the Republic of Belarus, were exposed to the influence of radioactive elements, in particular, Cs-137, far before the Chernobyl disaster (more than 20 years).

There was even a scientific prognosis of this radionuclide content in the foodstuff for the inhabitants of this area before 2000 [40]. The accident at the fourth power unit of Chernobyl nuclear power plant in 1986 has led to that no less than 180 million Ci of radioactive materials (excluding the activity of several tons of nuclear fuel, ejected close to the nuclear power plant) were released in the atmosphere. Radioactive nuclides of iodine-131, cesium-137, -134, strontium-90, and plutonium-239 contaminated a vast territory of the Republic of Belarus, Ukraine, Russia and other European countries [43]. The levels of their contents in foodstuff, even by the official standards, are very high. Particularly in 1966, daily consumption of 9063.9-

14280.3 pCi of Cs-137 in foodstuff was considered to be acceptable for the inhabitants in the Gomel region [40].

The demographic situation in the Republic of Belarus before the contamination with radioactive cesium was favorable. The birth rate was significantly higher than mortality (even in the period of difficult post-war years). During the postwar period in Belarus, the maximum natural population increase of 17.8‰ were registered in 1960. However, since 1965, steady reduction in the birthrate with increase in mortality of population occurred. In 1985, the index value of natural increase of population only amounted to 5.9‰. After the Chernobyl accident in 1986, the demographic situation worsened to such an extent that since 1993, mortality in the Republic of Belarus has come to exceed the birth rate, and the rate of natural population growth has become negative [41]. The progressive decrease in birth rate and increase in mortality rate led to the fact that the value was -4.9‰ in 1999, -5.9‰ in 2002, -5.5‰ in 2003, and -5.9‰ in 2005 [41, 42, 50].

During the period from 1994 to 2008, the population of Belarus declined by 607.4 thousand (almost 5.9%), and at the beginning of 2009, it amounted to 9,671,900. Reduction in the number of children under the age of 15 years should be noted: during the period from 2000 to 2009, reduced by 290,000 [53].

The statistical data of the Ministry of Health-guard indicate quite unfavorable conditions of the health of inhabitants in the Republic of Belarus. During the period from 1990 through 2004 in most of the regions of the Republic of Belarus and in the city of Minsk, there has been registered progressive increase in the number of children with congenital defects [44]. Exceptional cases consist of Grodno and Vitsebsk oblasts (Table 1.1.1.). However, in these regions during these years, there has been a sharp decrease in the birth rate, indicating a large reduction in human reproduction (birth rate has declined from 13.2 to 7.8‰ in the Vitebsk region).

During the period from 2000 through 2008 in the Republic of Belarus, the cases of childbirth with congenital malformations and anomalies of development have increased from 359.5 to 558.7 per 100 thousands newborn infants [50-55].

Increased frequency of congenital malformations, with decrease in the birth rate, indicates an extremely difficult situation appeared in the reproduction of population in the Republic of Belarus. Taking this into account, as well as the progressive increase of mortality rate of

Table 1.1.1. The relative number of children with congenital malformations, identified for the first time (per 100,000 live births).

Name of the oblast	1990 year	1999 year	2003 year	2004 year
Brest	59.5	128.0	115.9	86.2
Vitsebsk	48.3	50.3	—	39.9
Gomel	38.9	70.6	—	86.8
Grodno	72.7	91.0	—	45.9
Mogilev	52.1	80.5	—	90.7
Minsk	57.3	104.5	—	140.2
Minsk city	92.2	128.8	240.5	217.1

the population, we can mention about the origin of the demographic catastrophe. If the decrease in fertility rate could be explained to the inhabitants who does not know the true picture of the state of their health, as lacking motivation to give birth to children, but not as their inability to have children (the latter case happens much more frequently), then there could not arise any objection against the statistic data about the number of children with congenital defects.

The epidemiological situation for congenital defects in the present Belarus is such that it is no longer possible for specialists with high academic ranking to discuss in two ways. About the increasing number of births with congenital malformations in the Republic of Belarus, especially in the regions affected by the Chernobyl catastrophe, we can make only one unequivocal conclusion. And such a conclusion was made by the staffs of this institution in the official scientific reports [35, 36, 37].

This conclusion does not suit the nuclear lobby and their representatives of the former Soviet Union, specifically, in the Republic of Belarus. They have closed the Institute of congenital and hereditary diseases created even in the USSR, led by an outstanding scholar and geneticist, professor of teratology, G. I. Lazyuk, which was the unique research organization that, for many years, conducted extensive scientific research for the problems of the congenital pathology of human being, including statistical analysis of the current situation. Currently, there is no academic structure in the Republic of Belarus, competently answering the questions concerning the causes of occurrence of congenital pathologies. Thus, the academic schools created through several generations of scientists perished. Authorities ignorant of the medical science are in favor of those in power, in this case, in favor of nuclear lobby.

It is hardly to be surprised, because the International Atomic Energy

Agency at the UNO - the IAEA has long dominated the WHO — World Health Organization, imposed it on the agreement for non-disclosure of data on the effect of radiation on human health in 1959. Is it possible that this agreement more important than the health and lives of all of people on the Earth?

Officially registered congenital anomalies are just the upper tip of iceberg of the intrauterine developmental disorders that occur in the inhabitants having been in long-term contact with radioactive elements. It is impossible but to consider that the development of organisms of infants and the formation of their organs and systems in the conditions of constant exposure to Cs-137 and other radioactive elements inevitably lead to dysfunction of the organisms in their adult stages.

And here, it is worth referring to the high mortality rate of adults by sudden cardiac arrest, the real causes of which lie, in some cases, in disturbance of the formation of structural elements of the organ in the prenatal and postnatal ontogeny. Some of these conditions can be recorded in children with failure of the electro-physiological process of the myocardium. It is defined that there is dependence between the frequency of their occurrence and the concentration of Cs-137 in the organism [45, 46, 47].

In childhood, this pathological process is not a direct cause of lethal outcome. However, it may substantially afflict the clinical course of other diseases. As an example, we can point to the death of a baby from the Chernobyl zone due to viral infection, accompanied with development of heart failure, whose cause of death was not only the direct influence of viral agent on the heart, but also the influence of radioactive nuclide Cs-137 incorporated into this organ. Unfortunately, the effects of radiation factor are absolutely not considered for the occurrence of the pathological process, as an inductor of disorders of the cardiovascular system, as well as of the immune system.

Considering the extreme urgency for the inhabitants of the regions affected by Chernobyl catastrophe, which are problems of their reproduction in this section, analyses are implemented of results from clinical, experimental and radiometric investigations conducted by the author, who directed, from 1990 to 1999, members of Gomel State Medical Institute, being devoted to the impact of incorporated radionuclide Cs-137 to the process of reproduction.

As in the previous publications [3, 5, 6, 7], the author shares the methodological approaches, on the basis of which these researches were carried out:

1. Assessments of medical and biological effects taking into account the measured amount of radionuclides incorporated into the organism;
2. Clinical studies on the pathological processes, and modeling it in the experiments on laboratory animals (clinical and experimental approach);
3. Studies on the structural, functional and metabolic changes occurred throughout the whole organism as well as in the individual organs and systems;
4. Assessments of the degree of severity of pathological conditions from the viewpoint of disorders in the integrative processes of the organism, which enables to link together the pathological changes occurring in various organs.

Chapter1.2. § Female reproductive system in condition of incorporation of radio-cesium

On describing the pathology of intrauterine development of embryo caused by the influence of incorporated radio-cesium, it is necessary above all to refer to the condition in the female reproductive system. The vulnerability of the female reproductive system to the radioactive emission is shown in numerous scientific studies more than 30 years ago [9]. However, the current ecological situation compels to conduct the analysis of the state of this system in condition of long term exposure to radioactive elements incorporated into the organism. In this relation, we made assessments of health condition of women in reproductive age, considering the production of gonadal hormones and the levels of radio-cesium in the organism.

When the quantitative level of incorporation of Cs-137 in the female organism goes beyond 40 Bq/kg, hormonal inversions were revealed in various phases of the menstrual cycle, and it naturally caused disruption of the menstrual cycle. In particular, increase in the level of progesterone and decrease in the level of estradiol were recorded in the first phase, while in the second phase decrease in the level of progesterone and increase in the level of estradiol were recorded (Figures 1.2.1, 1.2.2, 1.2.3, and 1.2.4).

These hormonal changes lie in the basis not only of the disease of female genital sphere, but of the causes of infertility, because, in these

Fig. 1.2.1. The level of estradiol in the first phase of the menstrual cycle.

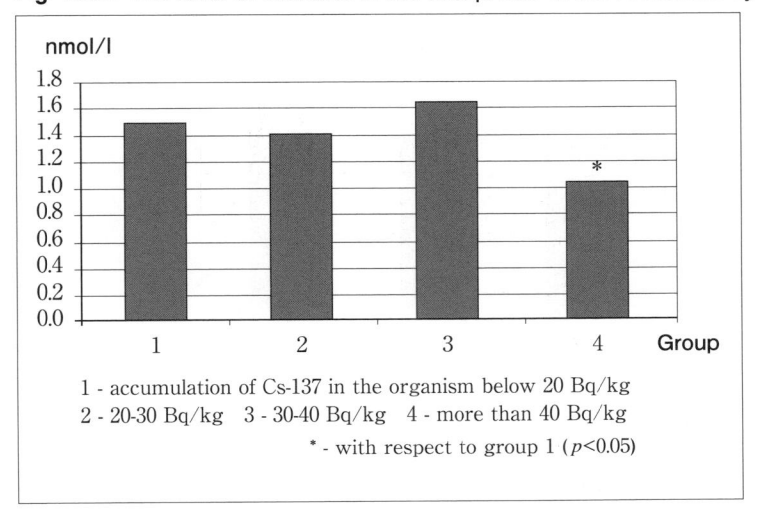

1 - accumulation of Cs-137 in the organism below 20 Bq/kg
2 - 20-30 Bq/kg   3 - 30-40 Bq/kg   4 - more than 40 Bq/kg
* - with respect to group 1 ($p<0.05$)

Fig.1.2.2. The level of progesterone in the first phase of the menstrual cycle.

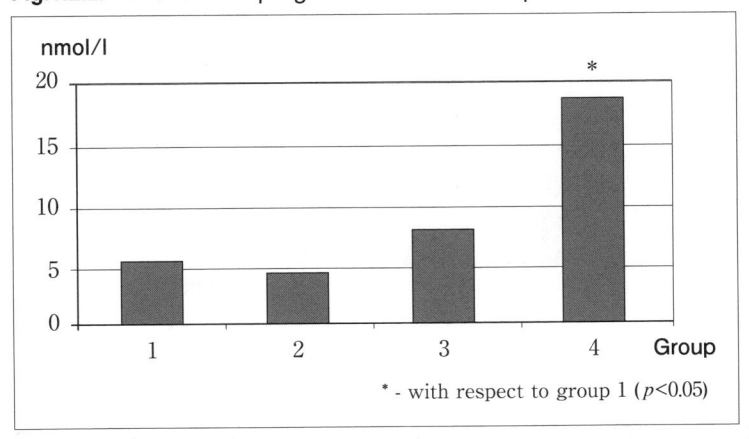

* - with respect to group 1 ($p<0.05$)

conditions, the uterine mucosa as well as the genital tract are not prepared for the process of fertilization and interactions with the embryo [34].

These were confirmed by the experiments in laboratory animals (non-purebred white rats), when the average content of radionuclide Cs-137 in the organism was 54.30±6.28 Bq/kg (in control, 14.05±3.31 Bq/kg), the blood progesterone level was found to be decreased as compared with that of the control group, in the estrus stage −23.96±6.94 nmol/l, (in control

Fig. 1.2.3. The level of estradiol in phase II of the menstrual cycle.

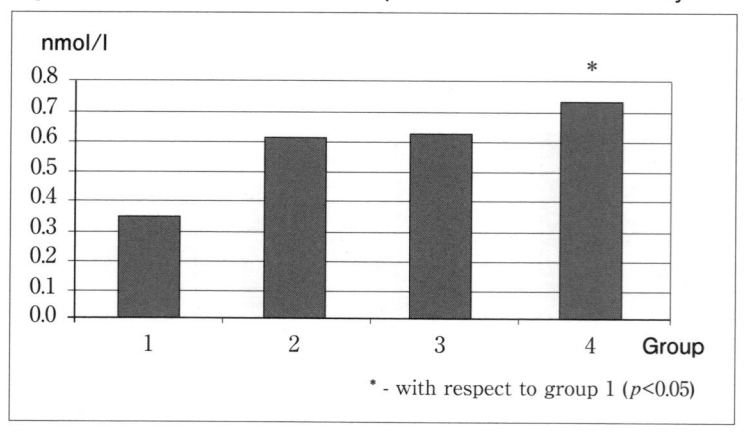

[Bar chart: nmol/l vs Group. Group 1 ≈ 0.35; Group 2 ≈ 0.61; Group 3 ≈ 0.62; Group 4 ≈ 0.73*]

* - with respect to group 1 ($p<0.05$)

Fig. 1.2.4. The level of progesterone in phase II of the menstrual cycle.

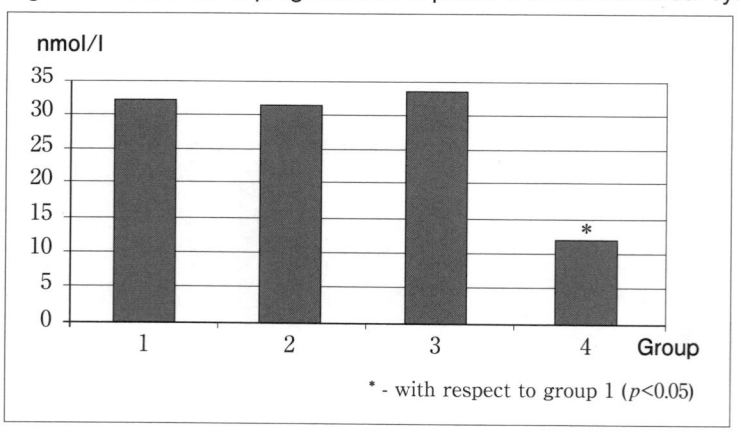

[Bar chart: nmol/l vs Group. Group 1 ≈ 32; Group 2 ≈ 31; Group 3 ≈ 33; Group 4 ≈ 11*]

* - with respect to group 1 ($p<0.05$)

— 61.01±15.66 nmol/l) and the uterus was decreased in the wall thickness — 13.91±0.99 conventional unit (in control — 16.57±0.52 conventional unit). Meanwhile, the ovarian data of these animals revealed no significant reduction in the number of follicles of various stages of development, including the secondary stage in comparison with the controls [34].

However, a number of authors indicate that suppression of oogenesis occurs at the combined impact of I-131 and Cs-137 in sufficiently large quantities [2]. In this case, in long-term observation (for 6 and 12 months), the destructive processes in the ovaries are intensified, resulting in reduction in the total number of follicles by 53%. And, under the influence incorporated radio-cesium, pronounced hormonal changes occur in the female organism, affecting various linkages of neuro-hormonal regulation, indicated by the research conducted by Yagovdik I. N. [29].

It is shown that log-term impact of radio-cesium incorporated into the organism of young female promotes disturbance of their hormonal homeostasis, that is, relative or absolute hypo-progesteronemia (reduced levels of progesterone in the blood) with a background condition of hyper-estrogenemia (increased levels of estrogen in the blood) and hyper-testosteronemia(increased levels of testosterone in the blood).

This appears particularly apparent at a concentration of Cs-137 above 50 Bq/kg. In this case, each of the sixth women is lacking ovulation. Thus, under the influence of incorporated radioactive cesium, there occurs inadequacy of luteal phase of the menstrual cycle and anovulation, reflecting disturbance of the hormonal regulatory processes.

In final conclusion, this results in infertility, as one of the main, in our opinion, causes of reduction in the birth rate in the territories contaminated with radionuclides. Investigations devoted on the formation of female genital system in the condition of long-term incorporation of radioactive cesium elicit great interest.

Girls living in conditions of chronic exposure of radioactive nuclides (level of Cs-137 contamination of the living territories − 15-40 Ci/km^2) are behind in the development of internal genital organs, with retardation of development of the secondary sexual characteristics (37% of those surveyed) and disorder of menstrual cycle (81% of those surveyed). In 39% of the girls, disorders of the gonadotropic pituitary function are noted, and in 31.5% of the cases, steroid-genesis (disturbance of biosynthesis of gluco-corticoid hormones). The obtained results indicate depression of the endocrine system, and thereby disturbance in the regulation of reproductive function.

Relationship between the degree of disorder of sexual maturation and the level of radioactive exposure are revealed [32]. The clinical observations were confirmed by the experiments with laboratory animals. Dietary intake of the radionuclide Cs-137 into the maternal organism in a period of pregnancy results in disruption of the development of the genital organs of offspring. In particular, in the ovaries of individuals in pubertal period of development, significant reduction in the number of mature follicles and increase in the number of atretic form were revealed in comparison to controls. There was a simultaneous existence of mature follicles and functioning corpora lutea. In these animals, delay in formation of the mucosal membrane of the oviducts and uterus occurred.

Severity of the above-mentioned changes were in direct dependence on the amount and duration of intake of radionuclide Cs-137 into the organism from food product [33].

Chapter 1.3. § Male reproductive system under the condition of incorporated radio-cesium

Unfortunately, medical science does not have complete information of the influence of incorporated Cs-137 into organism for the status of male genital system. On the other hand, impact of external ionizing radiation on the status of this system is investigated in detail [9, 14, 24].

Male germ cells are sensitive to the ionizing radiation. Irradiation of relatively low intensity of 0.15 Sv can cause transient azoospermia. Complete sterility of 100% in male individuals develops with a single irradiation at a dose of 6 Sv and above.

Sensitivity of the male germ cells depends on the intensity of their proliferation and degree of differentiation at the moment of irradiation. The proliferating spermatogonia is particularly vulnerable to ionizing radiation, while the spermatocytes are less vulnerable, and the spermatogenic cells are still less sensitive (Fig.1.3.1).

With conservation of viability of the stem spermatogonia, spermatogenesis after irradiation can be restored to some extent.

It should be emphasized that the effects of irradiation to this system are assessed primarily on such criteria, as fertilizing capability of individuals and the status of offspring throughout several generations.

In long-term periods (1, 3 and 6 months) after irradiation to male rats at a dose of 3 Gy, reduction in the content of spermatozoa in the epididymis, in the content of nucleic acid and protein in the testis was observed. At the same time, fertility of the animals was substantially decreased [12]. Such results were obtained by Zolotukhina V.N. and Vuts V.G. [19] with general fractionated irradiation to male rats in 3 days course at a total dose of 75 rad (25 rad per day), as well as by Gladkova A.I. et al. [15] with X-ray irradiation to male rats at doses of 0.25 and 0.75 Gy. In the latter case, increase in the number of abnormal gametes was noted.

In the experiments on mice line of VAaVC and SVA, increase in pre-

Fig.1.3.1. Scheme of spermatogenesis.

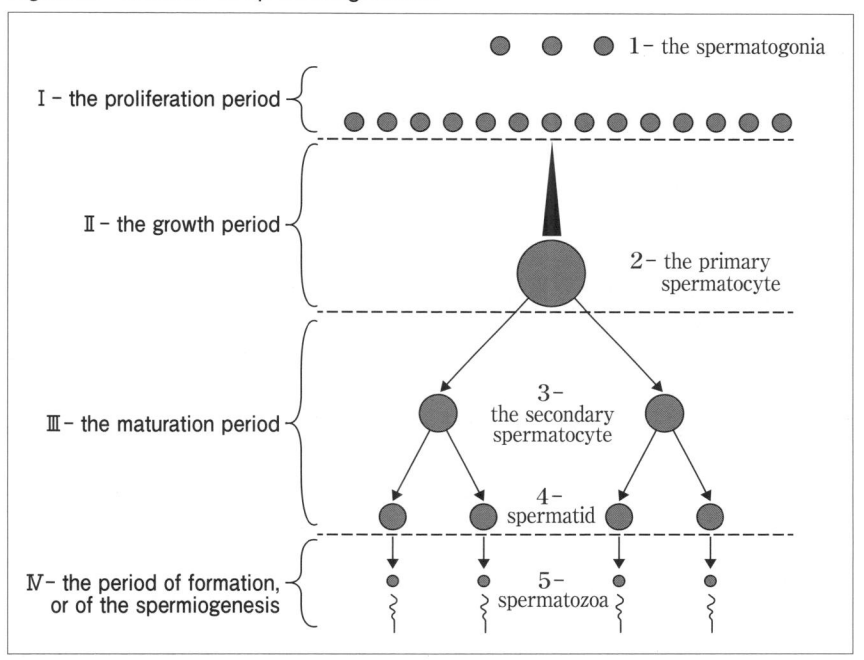

```
I - the proliferation period      ● ● ●    1 - the spermatogonia
                                  ●●●●●●●●●●●●●●

II - the growth period
                                         ●   2 - the primary
                                                 spermatocyte

III - the maturation period          ●   3 -        ●
                                       the secondary
                                       spermatocyte
                                    ● ●   4 -   ● ●
                                        spermatid

IV - the period of formation,       ↓ ↓         ↓ ↓
     or of the spermiogenesis       ● ●   5 -   ● ●
                                        spermatozoa
```

implantation death of embryos was observed, when fertilization occurred by the spermatozoa situated at the moment of irradiation at doses of 0.1-1.0 Gy on the stages of spermatogonia and stem cells [24].

The fertilizing ability of male individuals is associated primarily with the production of hormones that regulate sexual function and the formation of sperm. The endocrine part of testis is under the control of gonadotropic hormones, such as the pituitary follicle-stimulating hormone (FSH), which acts on the spermatopoietic epithelium, and the luteinizing hormone (LH), which stimulate the projection of testosterone by Leydig cells.

Testosterone directly affects the state of stem cells, while FSH promotes mitotic division of the spermatogonia and completion of spermatogenesis.

Suppression of production of sex hormones is shown under the influence of external and internal radiation exposure [3, 6, 9]. The most sensitive to radiation exposure is the evolving genital system. In this regard, the investigations conducted by the staffs of Grodno Medical University is interesting, which revealed negative influence of radionuclide Cs-137 on the formation of male genital systems in laboratory animals during the periods of antenatal and postnatal ontogenesis, leading to disturbance of production of testosterone and spermatogenesis [38].

However, radionuclide Cs-137 damages the germ cells themselves, with emergence of their structural and functional changes, changes in the structure of the genome should also be considered.

Chapter 1.4. § Mutagenic effects of radio-cesium.

A single oral administration of Cs-137 to male rats at a dose of 27 kBq/g, caused after 210-230 days statistically significant increase of univalents and chromosome fragments in the germ cells. At mating of these animals with intact females, increase in intrauterine (pre-implantation and post-implantation) death of offspring occurred [13]. The authors expressed an assumption that these effects are related to the influence of the genome pathologically modified by the internal environment of organism.

Similar results were obtained in the study of reproductive function of female mice of CC57W / MY line, whose two generations were in the environment of vivaria in Chernobyl and Kiev. At pairing Chernobyl females with intact males, reduction by 20-30% of the number of litters and neonates, and increase in pre-implantation death of offspring were noted [27].

In the offspring of rats, constantly being in the 30 km zone of Chernobyl atomic power plant, high frequency of structural abnormalities of the chromosomes of cells in the bone marrow, in the form of interstitial deletions, and other two-hit aberrations: dicentrics, rings, and translocations were recorded [20].

Investigations conducted by R.I. Goncharova and N.I. Ryabokon [16, 17] showed that feeding male laboratory mice with food product grown on territories contaminated with radionuclides, with achievement in the organism of radio-cesium concentration of 853 and 1103 Bq/kg resulted in increase in the level of chromosomal and genomic mutations in the genital cells and cells of bone marrow.

Such kinds of investigations in human population through years after Chernobyl catastrophe have not brought significant scientific results. In most of them, it was not able to identify the influence of incorporation of radio-cesium on the frequency of Mendelian pathology and multi-factorial congenital developmental defects [11, 21, 23].

However, the following was established that, in children resettled in the Minsk city from the districts of Gomel oblast contaminated with radionuclide Cs-137 in 7-8 years, increase in frequency of chromosomal aberrations in the form of dicentric and ring chromosomes, known as unstable indicators of radiation exposure was observed in the lymphocytes of peripheral blood [1, 11, 35].

In the post-emergency period, a growing number of developmental deformities occurred throughout Belarus, to a great extent, associated with increase in frequency of multiple deformities of development, reduction deformity of extremities and polydactyly, i. e., developmental deformities with a significant contribution of dominant mutations of DE NOVO.

Analyses of the frequency of isolated and multiple congenital malformations in children born between 1987-1998 showed excess of these rates in the districts with contamination level of 15 Ci/km^2, as compared with controls [36, 37]. The authors in these reports considered only contamination with Cs-137 in the soil of region and average values of doses received by the population, but not actual load doses of Cs-137 in the parents and their children. It should be noted that, in the same village, significant differences were observed in accumulation of radio-cesium among the inhabitants, depending on social and living conditions, cultural levels, and the state of food products consumed. Among children of Hilchiha and Ner villages, born in 1986 and 1987, levels of accumulation of Cs-137 and Cs-134 ranged from 1773.6 Bq / kg to 69.8 Bq / kg. Naturally, the radiation load doses among them are different.

Chapter 1.5. § Features of incorporation of radio-cesium in the periods of pregnancy and lactation.

Accumulation of radio-cesium in the organism is complicated and at present, a poorly investigated process. Previously, we showed that its intensity depends on gender, age, physiological condition of the organism, structural and metabolic features of the organs and tissues, and even on a group of rhesus surface antigen [3, 5, 6]. In particular, the female organisms accumulate radio-cesium in smaller amounts than males with identical nutritional conditions (Fig.1.5.1).

However, during pregnancy - a special physiological condition, an intense absorption of this radionuclide occurs in the gastrointestinal tract. In

Fig. 1.5.1. Accumulation of Cs-137 in the female and male organisms of experimental groups.

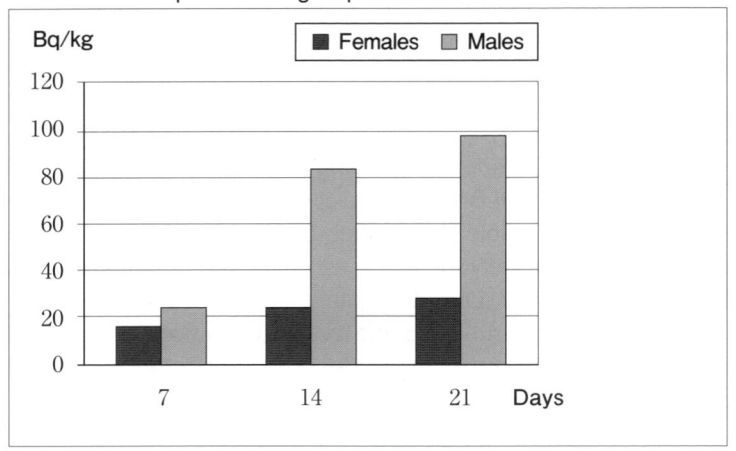

Fig. 1.5.2. Accumulation of Cs-137 in the organisms of mother and progeny in the experimental group for the suckling period.

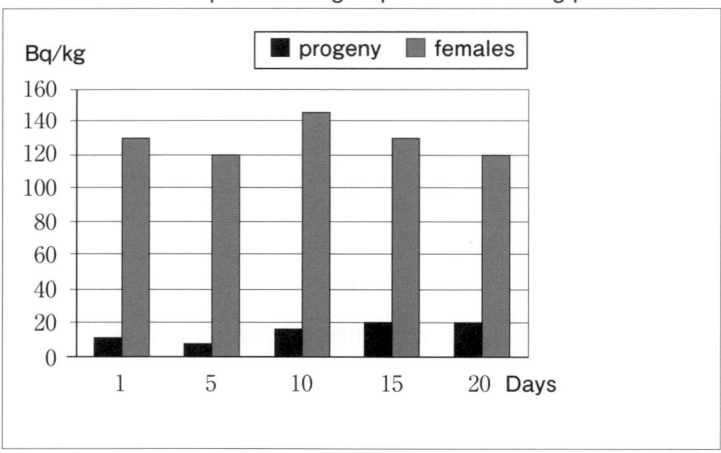

mammals, including animals and humans, to a great extent, it is absorbed by the placenta and it almost does not enter into the fetus (Fig.1.5.2). However, in the pathology of pregnancy and development of embryo, the concentration of radio-cesium in the developing organs can be significant [6, 8].

Possibly, hemochorial type structure in the placenta of human and a number of animals contributes to retention of this radionuclide. During the period of lactation, radio-cesium enters from mother to offspring with milk.

Table 1.5.1. Content of Cs-137 in the organism of the female rats and rat pups (Bq/kg)

Days after delivery	Experiment		Control	
	Females	Baby rats	Females	Baby rats
1-st	128.30 ± 6.52	36.64 ± 7.46	12.10 ± 7.59	3.95 ± 1.00
10th	34.46 ± 10.44	7.80 ± 1.53	8.53 ± 1.73	4.29 ± 1.36
20th	22.06 ± 6.23	9.69 ± 4.05	10.95 ± 4.20	6.29 ± 2.88
30th	19.32 ± 4.34	35.55 ± 5.92	18.74 ± 4.01	16.71 ± 2.49

In this case, the mother is exempted from it and the concentration in the organism is reduced, at the same time, it is increasing in the organism of children [5, 56].

In this respect, the results of experiments on laboratory animals (white rats) deserve attention, which were administered intra-gastrically aqueous solution of Cs-137 by 5 ml daily from the 10th to the 15th day of pregnancy. Animals in the control group received isotonic sodium chloride solution by 5 ml daily during the same period of pregnancy. Nineteen animals were used in the experimental group and 23 in controls. One hundred and fifty two and 224 cubs were obtained from them, respectively, which were conducted observations with registration of content of radio-cesium in the organism. It should be emphasized that the experimental and control groups were on the identical rations and in the same condition of maintenance.

Results of radiometric investigations are presented in Table 1.5.1. It shows that intake of Cs-137 at a period of pregnancy (10-15th days) led to the fact that, on the first day after delivery, its concentration in the female organism amounted to 128.70±6.52 Bq/kg, while that in the progeny was significantly lower 36.6±7.46 Bq/kg. After delivery and during a period of lactation, its content progressively decreased in offspring, as well as in the females. On the 10th and 20th days of life, radio-cesium levels in the offspring of the experimental group corresponded to those in the offspring of control group.

However, at the transition to independent feeding (after 20th day of life), increase in the content of this element was registered in the organisms of young rats in the experimental group, authentically larger than that in controls.

Thus, it can be stated that the animals subjected to the impact of Cs-137 in the period of intrauterine development, more intensively incorporate radio-cesium in food products, at the transition to independent feeding.

This fact requires further study, indicating us exclusive importance of the period of intrauterine development for subsequent existence of the organism.

Differences between female fetuses and male ones were not found in the incorporation of radionuclide Cs-137 in the placentas [39].

In our studies [5] it is revealed that people with Rh-positive blood type incorporate radio-cesium in larger quantities, in comparison to Rh-negative individuals.

Rh-negative women accumulated radio-cesium in the placentas significantly less (88.76 ± 12.37 Bq/kg, $n = 41$), than the Rh-positives (137.53 ± 12.98 Bq/kg, $n = 169$).

The same tendency was registered in young people in the Gomel city. Accumulation of Cs-137 in rhesus-negative individuals was 18.09 ± 3.88 Bq/kg ($n = 43$), while that in the Rh-positives was 23.81 ± 8.22 Bq/kg ($n = 182$). It is possible to assume participation of the antigenic determinant, representing Rhesus factor on the surface of erythrocyte, in the processes of incorporation of radio-cesium, considering the results of investigations about binding of this radionuclide to the membrane structures [25].

Chapter 1.6. § Pathology of the antenatal and postnatal development with incorporation of radio-cesium

1.6.1. Assessment of congenital defects in the human being with account of incorporation of Cs-137

There are scientific reports of an increase in the number of congenital developmental defects in the Republic of Belarus, as well as in the Gomel oblast in the post-Chernobyl period, while questions about the role of incorporated radio-cesium in teratogenesis were absolutely not considered [11, 21, 23]. However, presence of radio-cesium was registered in the dysplasia-centered lung tissue of fetuses from mothers living in the radiation zone [26].

Radiometry conducted among fetuses with congenital developmental defects and their placentas in a gestational period from 15 to 25 weeks, aborted for medical reasons in the medical institutions in the Gomel oblast, identified the presence of Cs-137 in them.

In this case, the content of this radionuclide in the placentas was higher than in the fetuses, 61.50±13.50 Bq/kg and 25.40±3.20 Bq/kg on average, respectively.

In embryos with congenital defects of the central nervous system, accumulation of radio-cesium in the placenta was still larger (85.40±32.70 Bq/kg). It should be noted that the investigated group mostly consisted of embryos with developmental defects, considered as multi-factorial origin, that is, arising as a result of joint effects of genetic and exogenous factors [22]. Congenital defects of the central nervous system were dominated, in particular, by anencephaly and spina bifida cystica (16 cases out of 42).

In children died on the first day after birth, from mothers who lived in a period of pregnancy in the Gomel oblast, significant accumulation of radionuclide Cs-137 was registered in their internal organs. In this case, histological investigations identified pronounced dystrophic and necrobiotic changes in the parenchymal cells of heart, kidneys, liver, and thyroid gland. The following examples support this conclusion.

Example 1.

Child A. was born with a weight of 950 grams, 38 cm in height. He died after 3 days and 20 minutes.

Clinical diagnosis – Intrauterine infection, Multiple organ failure, Premature birth.

Anatomico-pathological diagnosis – Intrauterine sepsis of unknown etiology. Morphological immaturity of the tissue structures of the lung, brain, kidney. Pulmonary atelectasis. Brain edema. Acute renal failure. Parenchymal dystrophy of the internal organs. General venous congestion. Premature birth. Extremely low body weight at birth.

Concentrations of Cs-137 in the internal organs are shown in Table 1.6.1.

Example 2.

Child D. was born with a weight of 750 grams, 34 cm in height. She died after 40 minutes.

Clinical diagnosis – Pneumopathy. Multiple organ failure. Premature birth. Extremely low body weight at birth.

Table 1.6.1. The concentration of Cs-137 in the internal organs

Organ	Concentration Cs-137, Bq/kg
Heart	5333
Liver	250
Lung	1125
Kidneys	1500
Brain tissue	3000
Thyroid gland	4333
Thymus	3000
Small intestine	2500
Colon	3250
Stomach	3750
Spleen	3500
Adrenals glands	1750
Pancreas	11000

Table 1.6.2. Concentrations of Cs-137 in the internal organs

Organ	Concentration of Cs-137, Bq/kg
Heart	4250
Liver	277
Lung	2666
Kidneys	1687
Brain tissue	1363
Thyroid gland	6250
Thymus	3833
Small intestine	1375
Colon	3125
Stomach	1250
Spleen	1500
Adrenals glands	2500
Pancreas	12500

Anatomico-pathological diagnosis – Pneumopathy - pulmonary atelectasis. Morphological immaturity of the tissue structures of lung, brain and kidneys. Brain edema. Parenchymal dystrophy of the internal organs. General venous congestion. Hemorrhage under the serous membrane. Premature birth. Extremely low body weight at birth.

The concentration of Cs-137 in the internal organs is shown in Table 1.6.2.

Example 3.

Child V. was born with a weight of 3500 grams, 51 cm in height. He died after 5 months and 12 days.

Clinical diagnosis - Enterosepsis of mixed etiology(salmonella typhi murium + staphylococcus aureus), septicopyemia form (bilateral focal confluent broncho-pneumonia, right sided pleurisy, acute enterocolitis). Fulminant course. Septic shock. Multiple organ failure. Immunodeficient state. Acute respiratory viral infection. Exudative-catarrhal diathesis. Rickets type II, subacute course.

Anemia of mixed etiology, moderate severity.

Anatomico-pathological diagnosis – Sepsis of mixed bacterial etiology (staph. aureus + salm. typhi murium "a" bacterial numbers of 386 - 389); Catarrhal enteritis, desquamative pneumonia, focal serous interstitial myocarditis, hepatitis, nephritis, splenomegaly, Hemolytic uremic syndrome. Bilateral serous fibrinous pleurisy. Brain edema. Granular and fatty degeneration of the hepatocytes, granular degeneration and necrosis of the epithelium of renal tubules. General venous congestion, fibrin thrombi and emboli in vessels; hemorrhage under serous membrane. Focal nodular sialoadenitis.

The concentration of Cs-137 in the internal organs is shown in Table 1.6.3.

Example 4.

Child A. was born with a weight of 1690 grams, 42 cm in height. He died after 3 days and 5 hours.

Clinical diagnosis – Pneumopathy. Intracerebral hemorrhage. Right-sided pneumothorax. Multiple organ failure. Premature birth.

Anatomico-pathological diagnosis – Bilateral massive intraventricular hemorrhage with tamponade of the lateral ventricles of the cerebrum. Pneumopathy and atelectasis, hyaline membrane. Pneumothorax on the right side. Brain edema. Parenchymal degeneration of the internal organs.

The concentration of Cs-137 in the internal organs is shown in Table 1.6.4.

Example 5.

Child K. was born with a weight of 3200 grams, 52 cm in height. He died after 10 days and 2 hours.

Clinical diagnosis – Multiple congenital developmental defects, congenital heart disease with pulmonary congestion, double cleft of hard and soft palate, stigma of dysembryoplasia(Rubinstein-Taybi syndrome). Bilateral lobular broncho-pneumonia, acute course, respiratory failure of III degree. Conjugated jaundice.

Table 1.6.3. Concentration of Cs-137 in the internal organs

Organ	Concentration Cs-137, Bq/kg
Heart	625
Liver	525
Lung	400
Kidney	250
Brain tissue	305
Thyroid gland	250
Thymus	1142
Small intestine	571
Colon	261
Stomach	1500
Spleen	428
Pancreas	1312

Table 1.6.4. Concentration of Cs-137 in the internal organs

Organ	Concentration Cs-137, Bq/kg
Heart	4166
Liver	851
Lung	1195
Kidney	2250
Brain tissue	90
Thyroid gland	1900
Thymus	3833
Small intestine	3529
Colon	3040
Spleen	1036
Adrenals glands	2500

Anatomico-pathological diagnosis - Multiple congenital developmental defects. Ventricular septal defect of heart, bilateral hydronephrosis, complete pass-through bilateral cleft palate. The syndrome of disseminated intra-vascular coagulation, bilateral fibrinopurulent polysegmental hemorrhagic pneumonia with foci of necrosis. Brain edema.

The concentration of Cs-137 in the internal organs is shown in Table 1.6.5.

Example 6.
Child Y. was born with a weight of 3970 grams, 55 cm in height. She died after 9 hours and 10 minutes.
Clinical diagnosis - Intrauterine infection. Multiple organ failure.
Anatomico-pathological diagnosis - Intrauterine infection (herpes), congenital pneumopathy, pleurisy, interstitial hepatitis, focal infiltration of the stroma of pancreatic gland, the kidney, swelling of the endothelium, hyperchromatism and intranuclear inclusion in the alveolocytes, the neurocytes,

Table 1.6.5. Concentration of Cs-137 in the internal organs

Organ	Concentration Cs-137, Bq/kg
Heart	1071
Liver	882
Lung	1500
Kidneys	812
Brain tissue	1693
Thymus	714
Small intestine	2200
Colon	4000
Spleen	2000
Adrenals glands	4750

Table 1.6.6. Concentration of Cs-137 in the internal organs

Organ	Concentration Cs-137, Bq/kg
Heart	1491
Liver	1000
Lung	2610
Kidneys	583
Brain tissue	714
Thyroid gland	1583
Thymus	833
Small intestine	590
Spleen	2125
Adrenals glands	2619
Pancreas	2941

the hepatocytes, and the renal tubular epithelium. General venous congestion. Parenchymatous degeneration of internal organs. Hypoxic encephalopathy.

The concentration of Cs-137 in the internal organs is shown in Table 1.6.6.

The presented examples indicate significant accumulation of Cs-137 in the internal organs of dead children. The clinical and anatomico-pathological diagnoses are presented in the form in which they appeared in the official medical documentation. Although pathologists exhibited various disease as causes of the death, it is possible to claim with confidence that, precisely, toxic effect of radio-cesium in a period of intrauterine development and after birth was the primary cause of death of the newborns.

Based on the results of radiometric investigation, in these cases, in our opinion, it is appropriate to speak of radiation-toxicity syndrome in fetus and newborn. And, just as without virological and bacteriological investigations, one can not make diagnosis of intrauterine infection, so without radiometry of the internal organs, one can not find the real cause of death of fetuses and neonates in radioactively contaminated territories.

1.6.2. Assessment of embryo-fetogenesis in laboratory animals at incorporation of radio-cesium in the period of pregnancy.

a) Experiments with white rats.

The aim of the study was to complete morphological and functional investigation of embryo-feto-genesis in non-purebred white rats at incorporation of radio-cesium with components of dietary ration [48].

One hundred and thirty seven pregnant female non-purebred white rats, 745 embryos and 344 rat pups were used. The day of detection of spermatozoa in the vaginal smears was considered the first day of gestation. Embryos were subjected to investigation on the twentieth day of intrauterine development, a day before the expected birth. Rearing and feeding of the rats were carried out in an environment of vivarium. Animals of the experimental groups received daily in the course of entire gestation, food products in the composition of — meat or grain with Cs-137 in concentrations of 5587 Bq/kg and 445.7 Bq/kg, respectively. Animals of the control groups received meat or grains, with concentrations of radio-cesium, 49.0 Bq/kg and 44.2 Bq/kg, respectively.

Considering the quantity of consumption of products, in accordance with the prescribed ration, animals in the first experimental group received 84 Bq of Cs-137 daily with meat, those in the first control group, 0.74 Bq of Cs-137, those in the second experimental group 16 Bq of Cs-137 with grain, and those in the second control group, 0.016 Bq of Cs-137.

Determination of the level of accumulation of Cs-137 in the animals of the first experimental and the first control groups was not carried out.

In females of the second experimental group, the concentration of Cs-137 by the end of gestation amounted to 132.77±10.77 Bq/kg, and that in females of the second control group, 9.22±2.90 Bq/kg, respectively. In the offspring born in the experimental group, concentration of radio-cesium in the organism was 6.47±2.18 Bq/kg, in the control group, 1.61±0.87 Bq/kg.

Numbers of females, fetuses and rat pups used in the experiments are presented in Table 1.6.7.

For the study of pathology in embryo-feto-genesis, animals in the experimental and control groups were decapitated on the 20th day of gestation after euthanasia with ether anesthesia. Fetuses were extracted from the uterus, to make their external inspection with purpose to identify developmental disorders, and measurements of their weight. One of the fetuses from each litter was fixed in the Bouin's mixture, and others in 96° alcohol. Numbers of locations of implantation, living fetuses in the uterus,

Table 1.6.7. Numbers of females, fetuses and rat pups used in the experiments

Group name	Embryo fetogenesis Number		Postnatal development Number	
	Females	Fetuses	Females	Rat pups
First experimental	20	115	4	69
First control	23	100	10	37
Second experimental	24	292	15	127
Second control	24	238	17	111
Total	91	745	46	344

and the number of corpora lutea in the ovaries were counted, calculating indicators of pre- and post-implantation death of embryos.

In the course of study, the following investigations were performed:
1. Investigation of the state of internal organs of fetuses of rats by the method of Wilson in modification by A. P. Dyban [18]. For this purpose, embryos fixed in Bouin's mixture were embedded in paraffin tables, and series of parallel sections were made with razor blades.
2. Investigation of the state of skeletal bones in rat fetuses. For this purpose, embryos fixed in 96° alcohol, were subjected to the process by the method of Dawson in modification of A. P. Dybana with coloration of the marker of bone ossification by alizarin red. The length of skeletons of embryos (parieto-coccygeal size) was measured with a compass, and the length of ossification marker of the individual bone was determined with assistance of ocular micrometer, binocular magnifier MBS-10;
3. In the blood of female rats of the first experimental and second experimental groups on the 20th day of gestation, contents of total bilirubin, urea, creatinine, total protein, phosphorus, triglycerides, cholesterol, albumin, glucose, alkaline phosphatase activity, alanine amino-transferase, and aspartate amino-transferase were determined, using the analyzer "Synchron" CX "Beckman" Co..

The obtained results were processed by the methods of statistical variation according to Student's test.

The results of conducted investigations revealed that the alimentation to the females white rats from the first day of gestation with food ration, comprising meat at a concentration of radio-cesium 5587 Bq/kg, causes significant increase in pre-implantation death of embryos, 2.27±0.52, vs.,

0.80±0.31 in control ($p<0.05$). Use to the pregnant rats of oat grains at a concentration of radio-cesium 445.7 Bq/kg, did not cause significant pre-implantation death of embryos. Indices of post-implantation death of embryos in the experimental groups did not differ from indices of the control groups. In the embryos of experimental groups, average length of the skeletal bones was significantly shorter in comparison to the corresponding control (Table 1.6.8.).

In the first and second experimental groups, the number of embryos with absence of ossification centers of metacarpal and metatarsal bones was larger than that in the control groups.

Investigation of the state of skeletal bones of embryos of the first experimental group revealed symmetric hypoplasia of the markers of ossification of all skeletal bones, bilateral absence of markers of ossification of the pubic bones, and absence of ossification centers of the second and fourth metacarpal bones, and second, third and fourth metatarsal bones.

An analogous investigation of the skeletal bones of embryos in the second experimental group showed significant bilateral reduction in the length of ossification markers in all skeletal bones, except for the fourth metacarpal bone, and the second and third metatarsal bones (in these parameters, difference between the second experimental group and the control group was not significant). It also revealed bilateral absence of ossification markers of the pubic bones, the second metacarpal bone, and the fourth metatarsal bone.

Length of ossification marker of the humeral skeletal bones in the embryos of the first experimental group is reduced, in comparison to the control indicator by 20-25%, of the femoral bone by 30%, and the sciatic bone by 55-60%. In the embryos of the second experimental group, the length of ossification marker of the humeral bone was reduced, in comparison to control, by 16-20%, the humeral bone by 25-27%, the sciatic bone by 43-54%.

In the females of the second experimental group on the 20th day of gestation, increase in the content of serum albumin 13.83±1.11 g/l, in comparison to control 10.50±0.93 g/l ($p<0.05$), and of calcium 1.87±0.18 mmol/l, in control 1.31±0.16 mmol/l ($p<0.05$) was observed. In other investigated metabolic indicators, significant differences among animals in the experimental and control groups were not found.

Administration of aqueous solution of Cs-137 to the female rats of Wistar line in the second half of gestation (10 to 15 days) led to the fact that content of this radionuclide in the organisms of newborn pups, ($n =$

Table 1.6.8. Indicators of the skeletal systems of rat fetuses in the experimental groups

Name of indicator	The first experimental group	The first control group	The second experimental group	The second control group
Length of Skeleton, mm	21.39 ± 0.48	24.70 ± 0.41	23.84 ± 0.39	25.55 ± 0.31
The number of embryos with absence of ossification centers of metacarpal and metatarsal bones, %	31.4	13.0	33.8	25.0

152, control $n = 224$) was significantly larger in comparison to control, on average 36.64±7.46 Bq/kg (in control 3.95±1.00 Bq/kg). This condition was accompanied by pathological changes in the internal organs of pups. In their hearts, inter-fiber edema, diffuse necrosis of the cardiomyocytes and their dystrophy were observed. In the liver, protein dystrophy of hepatocytes, enlargement of the space of Disse, and hyperemia in the central parts of lobules were registered. In the kidneys, destruction of the glomeruli, spasms of afferent arterioles, and drastically pronounced degeneration of the tubular epithelium were determined (Fig.1.6.1.). The same changes were discernible in the rat pups on the 10th and 20th days after birth in suckling period of their development. However, these pathological changes were particularly pronounced in the 30-day-old rat pups, which switched to independent nutrition and had significant accumulation of radio-cesium in the organisms (Table 1.5.1.).

Thus, the infiltration of Cs-137 into the organisms of pregnant rats leads to significant disruption of the processes of embryo-feto-genesis, which manifests itself in death of embryos at the stage of implantation in the mucous membrane of uterus, pathological changes of the bone systems in the form of hypoplasia of ossification markers in most skeletal bones, and dystrophic and necrobiotic changes of the cells in internal organs.

b) Experiments in Syrian hamsters.

The purpose of the study was to investigate influence of radionuclide Cs-137, incorporated in pregnant female Syrian hamsters, on the development of their embryos.

Twenty nine pregnant female Syrian hamsters with weight of 100-150

Fig. 1.6.1.

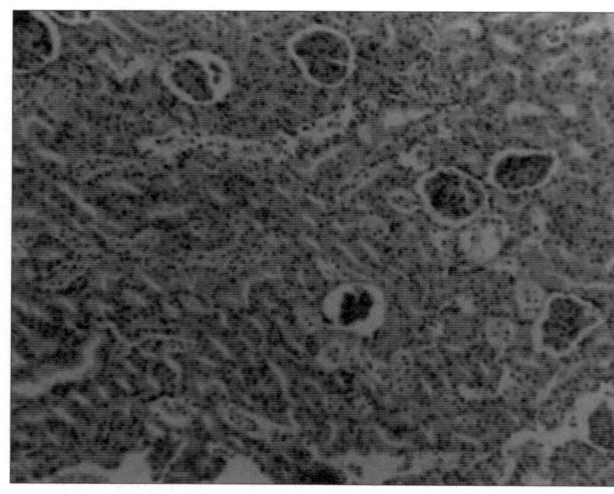

Histological structure of the kidney of the newborn rat with the accumulation of radio-cesium of 40 Bq/kg in the organism. Shrinkage and destruction of the glomeruli, protein degeneration and necrosis of tubular epithelium. Stained with hematoxylin and eosin. Magnification by125.

grams were used. Time of fertilization was determined by the presence of spermatozoa in the vaginal smears. Sterile aqueous solution of Cs-137 with 100 Bq of radiation activity in a volume of 1 ml was intraperitoneally injected to 18 females in the experimental group on the sixth and eighth days of gestation. Eleven animals of the control group on these days of gestation received intraperitoneal injections of physiological solution of sodium chloride of 1ml in volume. Registration of the content of Cs-137 in the organisms of animals in the both groups was performed on the 10th day of gestation using the radiometer RUG-2.

Study of the status of embryos was performed on the 15th day of gestation, the day before the expected delivery. In this case, the number of corpora lutea in the ovaries, and of locations of implantation in the uterus were counted.

Indicators of pre-implantation and post-implantation death of embryos were calculated. The weight of fetuses and placentas was determined. The weight of the placenta was evaluated with respect to the weight of fetus in the form of placental-fetal coefficient. After external inspection to identify gross defects in body structure of the embryos – congenital development defects, they were placed in Bouin's mixture or in 96° alcohol. The fetuses fixed in Bouin's mixture were subjected to investigation of the state of internal organs by the method of Wilson-Dyban [18], and those fixed in 96° alcohol were processed by the method of Dawson with coloration of the skeletal bones by alizarin red [18]. Two hundred and eight embryos of the experimental and control groups were investigated by means of all aforementioned methods.

Conducted investigation demonstrated that content of Cs-137 in the organism of animals in the control group ranged from 4 to 20 Bq/kg (12.4±1.7 Bq/kg on average). In this case, embryos with congenital developmental defects – exencephaly, craniocerebral hernia, cleft lip and cleft palate, anophthalmia, and micro-ophthalmia were registered in 46% cases of gestation (5 animals). These defects belong to the multi-factorial group, their occurrence, according to some researchers [22], depends on the presence of genetic predisposition in the parents, and the impact by environmental agents in a period of gestation. The aforementioned defects were detected only in 20 (20%) embryos from 101 embryos in the control group, examined on the 15th day of intrauterine development. The introduction of Cs-137 on the 6th and 8th days of gestation (the 6 - 9th days of gestation in Syrian hamsters are the period of organogenesis and placentation, one of the critical periods of embryo-genesis) led to the fact that, on the 10th day of gestation, its concentration in the maternal organism was 246.60 ± 20.10 Bq/kg on average. In the study of state of embryos on the 15th day of gestation, teratogenic and embryo-lethal effects should be stated in 100% cases of gestation. Of the 18 animals in the experimental group, death of all embryos was registered in 9 (50%) animals at the stage of organogenesis and placentation. This also shows the indicator of post-implantation death in the remaining 9 animals of this group, 5.9±1.0, while 1.6±0.4 in the control group ($p<0.01$). Embryos with congenital developmental defects were detected in 9 females (50% of the number of animals in the group). In a total of 107 embryos of this group, congenital developmental defects were detected in 63 embryos (59%); exencephaly, cranial-brain hernia, cleft lips and palate, micrognathia, microgenia, micro-ophthalmia, and anophthalmia (Fig.1.6.2.-1.6.5.). It should be noted that the body weight of embryos in the experimental group was not significantly different from the body weight of embryos in the control group (1.29±0.04 g vs. 1.49±0.10 g, respectively). The placenta-fetus coefficients in these groups also did not show significant differences.

Very unfortunately, during the time of conducted experiment, we did not possess devices enabling precise determination of content of radio-cesium in so small in weight and size of the objects, what embryos of Syrian hamster were. Therefore, we present only the extreme parameters of the content of this radionuclide. In the embryos of the experimental

Fig. 1.6.2.   **Fig. 1.6.3.**   **Fig. 1.6.4.**

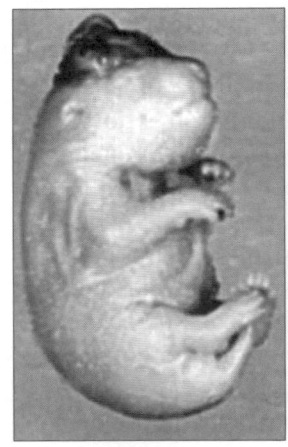

Exencephaly (absence of the bones of cranial vault), anophthalmia (absence of the eyes), on the 15th-day embryo of Syrian hamster in the experimental group.

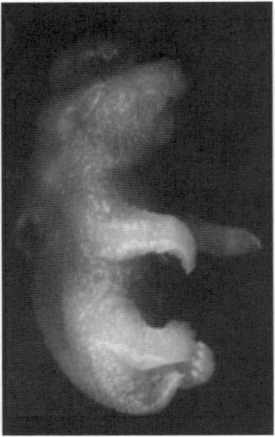

Exencephaly (absence of the bones of the cranial vault), microgenia (hypoplasia of the lower jaw), anophthalmia (absence of the eyes) in a 15th-day embryo of Syrian hamster in the experimental group.

Bilateral cleft lip and palate in a 15-day embryo of Syrian hamster in the experimental group.

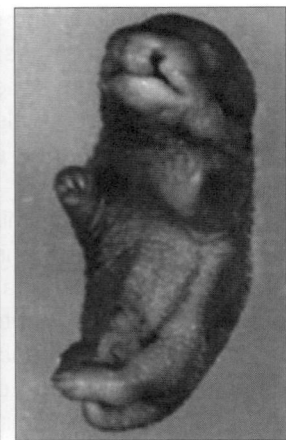

group, the concentration of Cs-137 was determined in the boundaries of 218-464 Bq/kg, and in their placentas within 511-2250 Bq/kg.

In the case of death of all embryos, concentration of Cs-137 in the uterus and embryonic tissue ranged from 426 to 1806 Bq/kg.

The data presented above showed that infiltration of radionuclide Cs-137 into the organism of pregnant animal - Syrian hamster, extremely adversely affects the development of embryos. In this case, congenital developmental defects occur, frequently registered in the human population [11], so-called multi-factorial. It is believed that the cause of their occurrence is a combination of genetic defects and impact of environmental factors [22, 23].

Impact of radionuclide Cs-137 in a relatively small quantity on the mother-embryo system provide condition for appearance of these defects, i. e., promotes phenotypical expression of defective genome in the animals originally containing it.

Based on the results of previous investigations, we intentionally injected radionuclide Cs-137 into female Syrian hamsters in the period of organogenesis and placentation (the 6th and 8th days of gestation), reaching such a concentration that would disturb metabolic processes in the organism, but would not cause the death of the animals. In all cases of the embryos, characteristic congenital developmental defects were

Fig. 1.6.5.
Skeletal bones

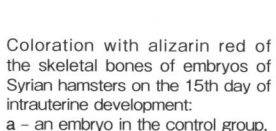

Coloration with alizarin red of the skeletal bones of embryos of Syrian hamsters on the 15th day of intrauterine development:
a – an embryo in the control group,
b – an embryo in the experimental group, absence of the bone of cranial vault, micrognathia (hypoplasia of the upper jaw), hypoplasia of the skeletal bones, stained with alizarin red.

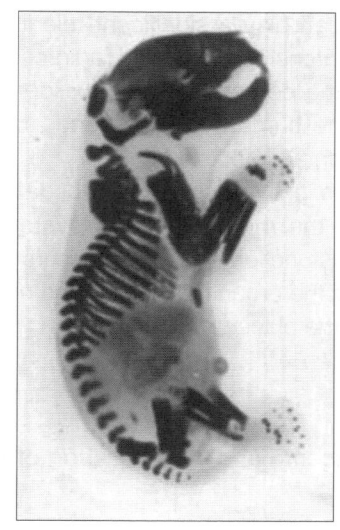

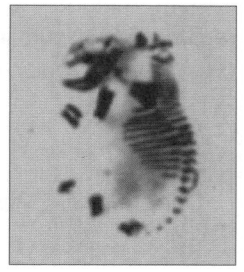

a   b

identified. In our opinion, metabolic discomfort, associated with cellular energy deficit arising in the mother-embryo system under the influence Cs-137 was the cause of congenital developmental defects of multi-factorial origin in Syrian hamsters. Impact of radionuclide Cs-137 on the processes of intrauterine development in white rats did not lead to emergence of these defects, however, was accompanied with disturbance in the development of embryo, demonstrating anti-metabolic effects in the form of hypoplasia of the ossification markers in a majority of the skeletal bones, and dystrophic and necrobiotic changes in the cells of internal organs. It should be emphasized that in the population of animals of white rats, embryos with multi-factorial congenital developmental defects were extremely rarely determined, while in the population of Syrian hamster, embryos with these defects were found constantly. The question is only about the frequency of occurrence of this phenomenon.

In the control group, they were isolated specimens, in the case of incorporation of Cs-137 into the mother-fetus system, the number of embryos with such a kind of developmental defects increased dramatically.

In this way, radionuclide Cs-137 causes in laboratory animals, disorders in the processes of embryonal development, the character of which are determined by the condition of genome. Damage to the structural components of placenta with disturbance in its endocrine and immunoregulatory functions can play a significant role in teratogenesis. It can be stated that the latter intensively captures radio-cesium

High levels of the content of radionuclide Cs-137 in the placentas were registered in the human embryos and animals with multi-factorial congenital developmental defects.

Considering the previously obtained data [3, 5, 6], one can make a conclusion that in the mother-embryo system in contact with radio-cesium, metabolic dysfunction syndrome occurs in which damage by this radionuclide occurs in the organs of mother and embryo and the provisional organs, in particular, the placenta.

Chapter 1.7. § Placenta and incorporation of radio-cesium.

The placenta is the most important provisional organ, providing development of the embryo. The placentas of human being and a number of mammalian animals, in particular, murine rodents have hemo-chorial type of structure. This means that a close relationship is established through the vascular system between the organism of mother and the developing embryonal structures. This relationship is regulated by the vital systems of both mother and embryo (endocrine, nervous, immune, and hematopoietic). However, the cellular and inter-cellular structures of the very placenta – representatives of extra-embryonal trophoblast – cytotrophoblast cells and syncytiotrophoblast cells play a special role in this process. They have a high level of metabolic activity, enabling them to perform many functions for the maintenance of intrauterine homeostasis. In particular, they provide infiltration to the fetus from the maternal organism through pino- and exocytosis and also through diffusion, of vitamins, and trace elements, substances without which normal growth, and development and differentiation of the organs and tissues of embryo is impossible [28].

The cells of cytotrophoblast provide execution of the endocrine functions of placenta by producing progesterone, estrogen, chorionic gonadotropin, chorionic somatotropin, chorionic thyrotropin and also chorionic luteotropin [28]. With the development of embryo and "aging" of placenta, the cells of cytotrophoblast transformed in syncytiotrophoblast, which is also biologically active. Particular attention should be paid to the participation of trophoblastic epithelium in the immunological relationship between the mother and fetus. It is considered to be proven that adsorption of maternal immunoglobulins, in particular, Ig M and Ig G occurs on the cytoplasmic membrane of trophoblastic cells [4].

Through the trophoblastic structure, the blood cells of maternal organism penetrate into the fetus and vice versa. It is proved that 30% of the erythrocytes of embryo are constantly circulating in the maternal blood, where the fetal lymphocytes are registered as well [4]. The fetus receives the immunocompetent cells and immunoglobulins from the maternal organism through placenta. In 1994, we proposed a hypothesis about the formation of immune systems in the developing organism through the maternal immunocompetent stem cells, passing through the placental barrier and forming humoral nexus of immunity [4].

The role of placenta in the transport of various chemical elements, including radioactive elements has been extremely poorly investigated. In this case, in the literature, there are directly opposite data about the transplacental transition of those or of other substances. This also applies to radio-cesium. Published results of the investigations conducted in laboratory animals - white rats, indicated limited infiltration of Cs-137, entering in the composition of food products in the maternal organism, to embryos [5].

Meanwhile, administration of aqueous solution of Cs-137 from the 10th to 15th days of gestation leads to more pronounced accumulation of it in the embryonal structures. In Syrian hamsters, radio-cesium infiltrates through placental barrier into embryos more intensively, than the results shown in the experiments presented above. In human being, radio-cesium also crosses through the placental barrier. In this case, it should be noted that the concentration of the radionuclide in the placenta is higher than that in embryos [8]. At the same time, significant accumulation of radio-cesium in the fetuses with congenital developmental defects may indicate a low level of the function of placental barrier. Accumulation of Cs-137 in the human placenta leads to its significant structural changes. With incorporation of this radionuclide at the concentration above 100 Bq/kg in the placental tissue, the number of intermediate villi increases toward the end of gestation, and the number of terminal villi decreases. The villi were covered with cytotrophoblast, and the stroma was coarse with a large number of connective tissue cells. Our attention was paid on a significant concentration of the syncytiotrophoblast in the terminal and intermediate villi, which indicated the processes of hormone formation.

In the placentas of these groups, pronounced disorders of circulation were observed in the form of hemorrhage in the stroma of villi and intervillous space, and small focal infarcts were determined.

Chapter 1.8. § Mutual endocrine relations in the mother-fetus system with incorporation of radio-cesium.

Incorporation of Cs-137 in the organisms of pregnant women is accompanied by pronounced hormonal changes in the developing embryo. The staffs of the Gomel Medical Institute conducted assessment of hormonal status of the mothers and fetuses in 74 cases of delivery, in which they were allocated into groups according to the content of radio-cesium in the placentas.

For example, the control group - absence of radio-cesium; the first group 1 - 99 Bq/kg; the second group 100 - 199 Bq kg; the third group - 200 Bq/kg and more of radio-cesium [39].

The conducted investigation showed that in the blood of fetus, the content of estradiol was significantly reduced, as the content of radio-cesium increased in the placenta. At the same time, the testosterone level increases significantly, and these tendencies were preserved not only in female fetuses, but also in male fetuses (Fig.1.8.1.).

In the maternal organism, reduction in the content of estradiol also occurs, as the content of radio-cesium increase in the placenta. The ratios of levels of estradiol in the mothers to those of estradiol in the fetuses in all groups were 0.9 on average. The ratios of levels of testosterone of the mothers to those of testosterone of the fetuses were reduced from 1.89 in the control group, to 0.49 in the third group. With the increase in the level of accumulation of the radionuclide in the placenta, more pronounced reduction in the ratio of estradiol/testosterone was observed in the fetuses. The level of progesterone in the blood of fetuses was significantly higher than that in the blood of the mothers. At the same time, both in the fetuses and mothers, a tendency of increase in the content of this hormone from the control group to the third group was observed.

In the maternal blood, a valid increase in the level of thyroid hormones – thyroxine and triiodothyronine, was identified, depending on the amount of radio-cesium in the placenta. In the fetal blood, irrespective of the amount of incorporated radionuclides, changes in the level of these hormones were

Fig. 1.8.1. The content of estrogen and testosterone in the umbilical cord blood of fetuses in the main and control groups

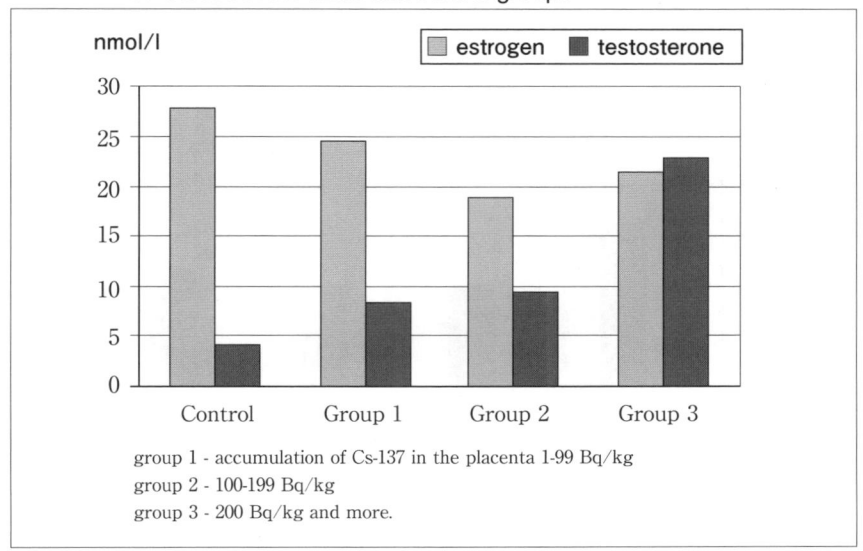

group 1 - accumulation of Cs-137 in the placenta 1-99 Bq/kg
group 2 - 100-199 Bq/kg
group 3 - 200 Bq/kg and more.

not observed.

It should be noted that a valid increase in the content of cortisol in the maternal blood occurred, with increase in the content of radio-cesium in the placenta, whereas the level of this hormone in the fetuses was reduced (Fig. 1.8.2.).

Thus, incorporation of Cs-137 in the mother-fetus system leads to significant hormonal changes, first of all, in the developing organism. It should be considered that the adrenal tissue intensively incorporates this radionuclide [6, 8, 49]. Incorporation of this radionuclide causes disturbance in the function of enzymatic systems of the mitochondria [47]. As a result, it can be assumed that the increase in production of male sex hormone, testosterone, and the reduction in female sex hormone, estradiol, are consequences of the impact of radionuclide Cs-137 on the hormone producing cells in the adrenal cortex. In this case, synthesis of cortisol - the main hormone of the cortex of adrenal glands suffers. This condition facilitates increased production of the pituitary adrenocorticotropic hormone, which stimulates the cells of the adrenal cortex, leading to overproduction of testosterone. A condition of congenital dysfunction of the adrenal cortex occurs, which will undoubtedly affect the subsequent development of the child. Inversion of the endocrine status of children in

Fig. 1.8.2. Content of cortisol in the blood of mothers and fetuses in the main and control groups

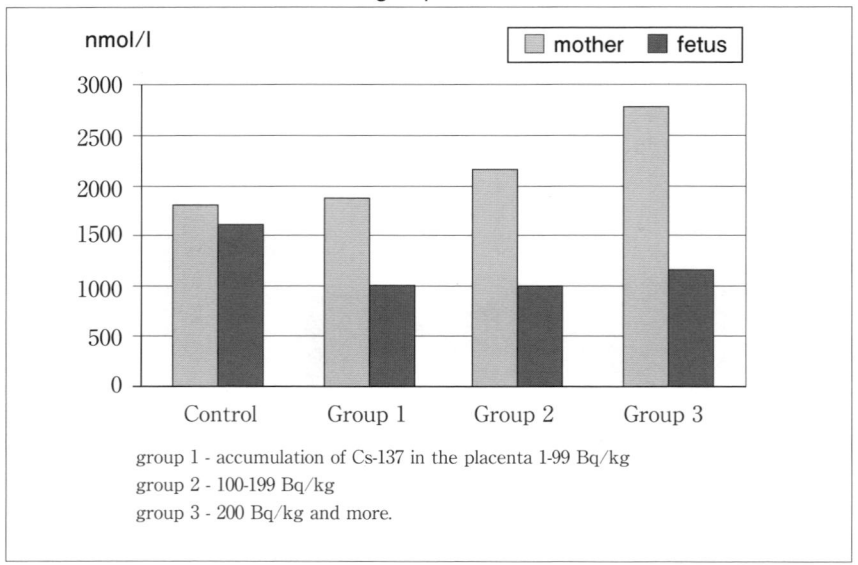

```
                                           □ mother  ■ fetus
nmol/l
3000
2500
2000
1500
1000
 500
   0
        Control      Group 1      Group 2      Group 3
```
group 1 - accumulation of Cs-137 in the placenta 1-99 Bq/kg
group 2 - 100-199 Bq/kg
group 3 - 200 Bq/kg and more.

a condition of impact of radio-cesium is, in our opinion, one of the main causes of disorders in sexual development, and in adaptation to conditions of external environment after birth, which lies in the basis of diseases of endocrine, nervous, immune and many other systems in the future.

Chapter 1.9. § Radiation-toxicity syndrome of fetus and newborn.

Radio-cesium - Cs-137 infiltrating into the organism, enters in interaction with numerous biological structures and, in particular, with a complex system, which is the mother-embryo system. Its impact on the maternal organism is implemented in the disturbances of:

The endocrine systems - including those with respect to regulation of sexual function;

The muscular system - changes in the tonus of the muscular tissue of sexual organs and vascular walls;

The cardio-vascular system - disturbance of the blood supply to uterus and to all of the organs with disturbances of their functions;

The nervous system - disturbance of functions with subsequent disturbances of neuro-regulatory relation with the developing embryo;

The immune system - reduction in the protective functions of the organism, which creates a condition for development of viral and bacterial infections in the mother-fetus system with subsequent characteristic of intrauterine infection. Disturbance of the integrative relationships in the mother-embryo system, leading to formation, in some cases, of congenital developmental defects and congenital immunodeficiency;

The urinary system - Renal lesions with subsequent delay in excretion of radio-cesium and toxins from the organism, which create conditions for disorders of intrauterine development of embryo.

The hematopoietic systems - At pronounced incorporation of the radionuclide, the number of erythrocytes decreases, which results in intrauterine hypoxia of fetuses and newborns.

The hepatobiliary system - a number of liver functions, which play leading roles in the metabolism of mother and fetus, are impaired. It is, first of all, the synthetic function, directed to the of formation of vitally-important substances for the organism, as well as, the ability to neutralize toxins, neurotransmitters, hormones, environmental agents alien for the organism. Regulation of protein, fat, carbohydrate and mineral metabolism is disturbed. Damage to the hepatocytes, and development of their fatty and protein degeneration, lead to disorders in metabolism of the mother-embryo system;

The reproductive system - Lesions of the ovarian structures, uterus, and oviduct, and as a consequence, disturbance of embryonal development.

Intrauterine development of the embryo - Infiltrating into the placenta, radio-cesium interacts with its structures - the vascular network (arterioles and capillaries) and the cells of trophoblast. In this case, disturbance of circulation, and changes in the production of hormones of the very placenta, and consequently changes in the endocrine system of mother and fetus occur.

Undoubtedly, the placenta restricts access of Cs-137 to the embryonal structures, as a fundamental barrier against it. In cases where the barrier for one reason or another is not effective, the radionuclide infiltrates into the embryonal structures, damaging them and causes congenital developmental defects.

Considering that Cs-137 dramatically reduces the energy potential of cells, and disturbs entire course of the metabolic processes, in particular, synthesis of the protein molecules, its involvement in the processes of teratogenesis is realistic enough. The experiment in Syrian hamsters is a vivid case in point. Under the impact of radio-cesium, a number of cases of developmental defects occur, related to a group of multi-factorial congenital developmental defect (malformations of the central nervous system, the facial part of the skull, and the heart). Their emergence is associated with the presence of certain genetic defects and the effect of provoking environmental factors [22]. If there is not a sufficient margin of safety in the genome, in the form of function of certain genes of individual alleles (parts of the genes do not function due to mutations), intervention of Cs-137 in the process of prenatal development completes formation of congenital developmental defects. In this case, radio-cesium acts as a provoker for the genetic defects inherent in the previous generations.

In this case, the dose of this incorporated radioactive agent should not necessarily be high. Action of radio-cesium, in on our opinion, is especially directed to destruction of regulatory relationship between the mother and embryos, including the participation of regulatory systems (immune, endocrine, nervous), maintenance of proper rates of synthetic processes and differentiation of the embryonal structures, necessary for realization of phenotypic features, under conditions of the aforementioned defects of the genome. In these circumstances, above all, anatomically complexly formed organs with, as a rule, long-term teratogenic termination periods - critical periods of embryogenesis (periods with the greatest sensitivity to various teratogenic impacts), the heart, the eyes, the central nervous system, the hard palate, and the external genital organs – are damaged (Fig.1.9.1.).

Considering that the frequency of genetic defects in human population increases from year to year, mainly due to radiation impacts, the significance of Cs-137 incorporated into the mother-embryo system, as an inducer of congenital developmental defects, increases. It must be considered that it can participate in teratogenesis, disturbing trophicity of primordia of developing embryos, directly influencing on the metabolism of embryonal cells and/or damaging the placental structure. It can especially clearly be seen in the formation of skeletal bones of the embryo. By reducing the intensity of proliferative processes in the rudiments of bone, radio-cesium causes their hypoplasia. It should be take into consideration that in conditions of progressive accumulation of this radionuclide, parallel deterioration of metabolic processes in the mother-embryo system occurs. In these conditions, the bone rudiments formed in later periods of embryogenesis (the bones of lower extremities) are affected more than the rudiments that are formed earlier (the bones of the upper extremities).

Fig. 1.9.1. Critical periods of human embryogenesis in weeks (Mur-Much, 1973)

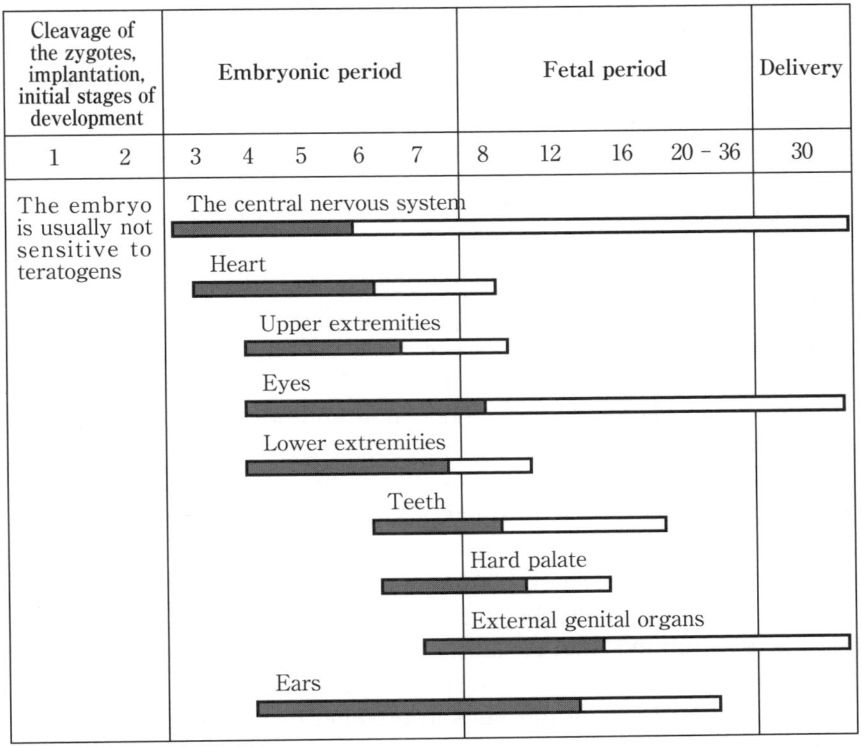

Cleavage of the zygotes, implantation, initial stages of development		Embryonic period					Fetal period				Delivery
1	2	3	4	5	6	7	8	12	16	20 - 36	30
The embryo is usually not sensitive to teratogens		The central nervous system									
			Heart								
				Upper extremities							
				Eyes							
				Lower extremities							
					Teeth						
					Hard palate						
						External genital organs					
				Ears							

Note. In the first two weeks of development, impact of teratogens usually leads to death of the embryo; from the third to eighth weeks - to major morphological abnormalities; from the ninth week in the embryo, as rule, physiological defects and minor morphological deviations occur.

Shaded areas – the most sensitive stage of the embryo to teratogens.

Areas without shading – stages with lower sensitivity to teratogens of the embryo.

We obtained similar effects by the simulation of oxythiamine-induced B1 avitaminosis in white rats and Syrian hamsters [57].

Except for congenital developmental defects, Cs-137 can cause death of the embryos.

Impact of Cs-137 on the maternal endocrine system particularly at the early stages of intrauterine development, distorts production of the ovarian hormones, resulting in which the uterine mucosa turns to be unprepared for the implantation of embryo. Infiltration of radionuclides into the oocyte, and fertilized ovum - zygote, dividing embryo - morula, and blastula, can cause in future, serious pathological changes in the developing embryonal structures.

Combination of genetic defects and inversion of endocrine status is very frequently observed.

Undoubtedly, defects in the genome of germ cells of both females and males, occur in the previous generations under the influence of all those radiological agents, and in particular of Cs-137, infiltrating into the organism. However, we certainly can not ignore the effects of chemical and biological mutagens.

Radio-cesium, influencing on the embryonal tissue in the fetal period, do not cause gross developmental defects, but has damaging effects on the cells of various organs. The pathological effects in this case can appear after birth. At this stage of embryonic development, as well as after birth, this agent causes damage to the highly differentiated cells of various organs, especially the immune, endocrine and nerve systems, and the heart, liver and kidneys.

The main path of entry of Cs-137 into the infant of lactation age is through the mother's milk or dairy products for artificial feeding. In the period of lactation, the maternal organism intensively eliminates radio-cesium, and therefore feeding children with this milk is unacceptable.

Therefore, it is impossible to agree with the PRL-99 of the Republic of Belarus, in which milk with contamination level of Cs-137 up to 100 Bq/kg (the permissible radiation levels-99) can be consumed.

Energy systems of the cells in growing organism are especially severely affected by the impact of this cellular poison. Diseases emerging in conditions of suppression of the endocrine status and the immune system, mostly infectious, mask the true cause of damage to the organisms of children – the effect of incorporated radio-cesium.

In this regard, for proper diagnoses of the pathological processes arising in newborn infants whose parents lived and/or live in the area of radiation contamination, it is necessary to conduct radiometric investigations on the children and mother for the identification of radio-cesium incorporated in their organisms.

For the purpose of setting etiopathogenetic diagnoses and consequently, for the purpose of proper treatments, the actual radiation-toxicity syndrome of the fetus and newborn caused by the impact of long-lived radionuclide Cs-137 on the mother-fetus system must be acknowledged, which we described earlier as one of the variants of incorporated long-lived radionuclides syndrome [3], in order to avoid errors in diagnoses and treatment of many diseases.

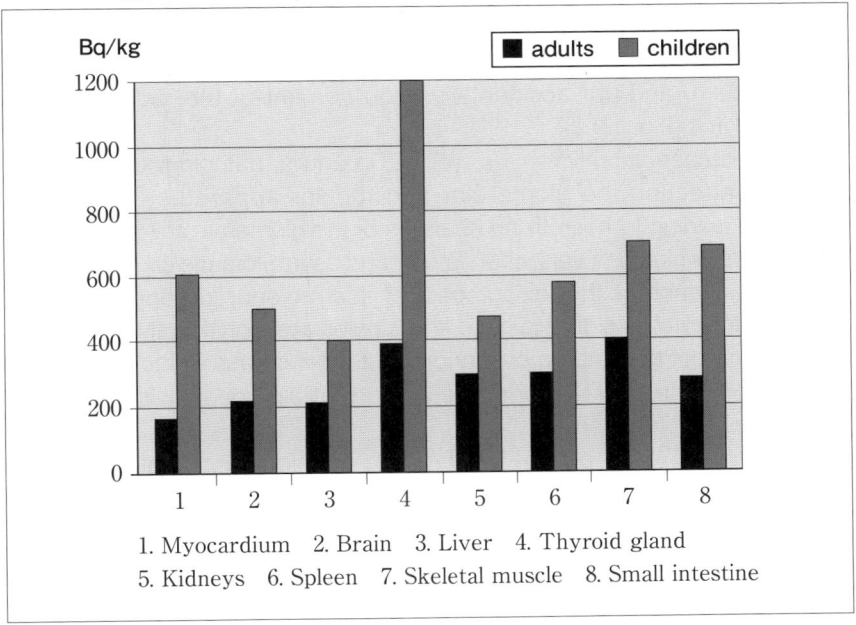

Fig. 1.9.2. Contents of the radionuclide Cs-137 in the internal organs of adults and children — inhabitants of the Gomel oblast, died in 1997 [6, 49]

1. Myocardium 2. Brain 3. Liver 4. Thyroid gland
5. Kidneys 6. Spleen 7. Skeletal muscle 8. Small intestine

Accumulation of Cs-137 was detected in the internal organs of dead children in older ages (Fig.1.9.2.). The high concentrations of the radionuclide in the thyroid gland, adrenal glands, pancreas, and myocardium are characteristic [49]. In histological investigations, the same pattern was observed, that in the fetuses and newborns - degenerative and necrobiotic changes in the cells of vitally important organs were for the most part incomparable with life. Lesion of the immune system - the cause of development of infectious diseases, is a documentary cause of death of the children.

However, undoubtedly, the impact Cs-137 causes lesion of the immune system, as well as of the cells of internal organs. In these conditions, even impact of the banal microflora will render extremely negative effect on the organism, and the distribution of tuberculosis, viral hepatitis receive widespread distribution in the human population. Lesion by radio-cesium of the immune system (first of all, its suppressor level) as well as of the parenchymal liver cells, causes, in conditions of the impact of infectious pathogen, burst of chronic hepatitis, difficult to treat with conventional methods. Hepatic encephalopathy, or hepatic failure, as consequences of toxic liver degeneration, cirrhosis or chronic degeneration of this organ, has become increasingly common.

The kidney is one of the excretory organs for radio-cesium out of the organism, and not accidentally, high content of the radionuclide is registered in it (Fig. 1.9.2).

In this case, in children, as well as, in adults, pathological processes develop, affecting the glomerular and tubular apparatus [5]. Vascular disorders, leading to necrotizing changes of the glomeruli, are the cause of renal failure, which has very often latent, and asymptomatic course. Uremia – a consequence of the toxic impact of this radionuclide appeared as if suddenly for clinicians. In this case, the tubules are significantly affected as well. It must not but to be mentioned about the increase in the Republic of Belarus for the recent years, of the number of individuals with neoplastic pathologies of this organ [30].

The heart - the one of the organs, functioning of which requires intense energy expenditure. In conditions of the impact of this toxicant, as Cs-137, it suffers as one of the first. The radionuclide at a concentration equal to 63.35 ± 3.58 Bq/kg in the organism of laboratory animals, caused reduction in the activity of creatine phosphokinase in the myocardial cells, the main enzyme of energy cycle, by 50%, in comparison to the animals whose concentration of Cs-137 in the organisms was 5.43 ± 0.87 Bq/kg [47].

Energy deficits, arising in relation to infiltration of the radionuclide into the cytoplasm of cardiac cells is the primary cause of disorders (reduction in the level) of anabolic metabolism, especially, synthesis of the protein structures involved in the contraction of muscle fibers. Processes of intracellular repair (renewal) in these conditions are dramatically disturbed Any of the stress (physical stress, neuropsychiatric impact, impact of toxic agents) can cause serious disorders in the operation of this organ, and of the entire cardiovascular systems with pronounced clinical symptoms. The latter is the dilated cardiomyopathy – sacciform expansion of the heart walls with loss of contractile ability, which occurs in individuals in ages of 30-50 years. The frequency of this disease increases from year to year. This is not by accident – more than 24 years have passed from the moment of Chernobyl tragedy, and children have grown, whose critical periods for the development of vitally-important including cardiovascular systems, occurred in the post-Chernobyl period.

Indicators of the adverse effects of radio-cesium on the heart are the disorders in the structures and functions of conductive system, regulatory processes in contraction and relaxation of the cardiac muscle. Even a small concentration of this agent can cause disorders in transmission of electric impulses through the conductive system in the form of various kinds of blocks. Relationship between the frequency of disorders of cardiac activities in children and the content of radionuclide in their organism was revealed [45, 46, 47].

In our opinion, explanation for this phenomenon again lies in the plane of understanding the existence of regulatory processes in the organisms of human being and animals, including regulation of the gene activity. External environmental factors which inhibit functions of the systems regulating (stimulating) the activity of genetic apparatus of the cells, will be inducers of occurrence of many diseases. In conditions of presence of the genetic defects, radio-cesium, inhibiting the energy processes in the cells of cardiovascular system, will block compensatory-adaptive processes directed to maintenance of vital activities of the organism, provoking the emergence of pathological processes.

With increase in the amount of radionuclide Cs-137 in the organism, frequency of disturbances of the cardiac function increases [7, 47], as well as, the severity of the lesion. Intensive death of the cardiomyocytes occurs. The result of this pathological process is the dilated cardiomyopathy mentioned above, and the sudden cardiac arrest.

Endocrine disorders in children have their origin in the period of intrauterine development. Hypoplasia of the adrenal glands, and the related insufficiency of hormonal production – consequence of the impact of radio-cesium in the intrauterine period. In the period fetogenesis and postnatal ontogeny, toxic damage to this organ and insufficiency of the production of hormones are observed. This is manifested most demonstratively in respect of cortisol production. The same can be said of the pancreas, gonads, and, of course, of the thyroid gland. Lesion of the last one is associated with I-131, as well as Cs-137. These two radionuclides have created a terrible situation for the health of the inhabitants, not only in the Republic of Belarus, but also in the Western Europe. The result was the high incidence of thyroid cancer and autoimmune thyroiditis. Contrary to the established views about the leading role of I-131 in the occurrence of these diseases, our findings approve that Cs-137 plays, in this case, no less important role, because it is intensively absorbed by the cells of thyroid gland. Eroding energetics of the cells of thyroid gland, it causes their death, disturbs cellular and intracellular repair, and differentiation of the cells, and moreover facilitates that structural components of the cells become antigens for the immune system. In addition, it affects the immune system, disrupting balance of the cellular populations (lesion of the suppressor level).

Immunological reactions occur, in which autoantibodies and immuno-competent cells do damage to the thyroid gland, with development of autoimmune thyroiditis, and from its background, and of cancer of the thyroid gland.

In connection with this, impact of radio-cesium on the thyroid gland should be considered from the perspective of disorders in the immune regulation of activities of the organs and tissue, as well as considering the nature of damage to cellular elements.

In conditions of the decay of short-lived I-131 with energy release destroying the structure of genetic apparatus in the cells, this causes relatively rapid development of the aforementioned pathological processes.

The immune system is exposed to the influence of Cs-137 in the period of intrauterine development. In this case, clinically and laboratory established immunodeficiencies occur, and the latent state manifests itself in the high frequency of allergic and infectious diseases. Intensive incorporation of this radionuclide in the organs of immunogenesis causes disturbance in the immunological and immunoregulatory relationship of the mother-fetus system, with emergence of pathologies of the intrauterine development (antenatal death, congenital developmental defects in the multi-factorial group).

In the postnatal ontogeny, incorporation of Cs-137 in the organs of immunogenesis creates conditions for chronic immune deficiency, which is one of the causes of development of the oncological and infectious diseases. It can not but to be mentioned about the increase in the malignant neoplasms of lymphatic and hematopoietic tissues in children [30].

The nervous system suffers from the impact of radio-cesium, starting from the period of intrauterine development. Malformations of the central nervous system occur under the influence of this radionuclide in human being and a series of experimental animals, in condition of the genetic predisposition (absence of activity in a series of the allelic genes), and refer to the multi-factorial group. Such malformations, as exencephaly, and craniocerebral hernia are most frequently observed. In the period of fetogenesis, impact of Cs-137 causes lesion of the volatile nerve cells capable of intracellular repair, and disturbance of formation of appropriate structures of the nervous system. The same effects appear at the incorporation of this radionuclide in the cells of nervous system in the postnatal ontogeny. In the cells of nervous system, in this case, drastic disturbance of metabolism of biologically active substances occurs [31]. In our opinion, intensive incorporation of radio-cesium in the structures of central nervous systems, is the cause of growing number of its malignant diseases, which was confirmed by the statistical data. For the period of 1992-2001, brain tumor occupied a leading position in the structure of oncological morbidity in children, living in the Republic of Belarus, along with the malignant neoplasms of lymphatic and hematopoietic tissue [30]. Proceeding from the aforementioned, Cs-137 should be considered as:

1. as a source of mutational processes in the somatic cells, which is one of major causes of increase in the malignant neoplasms;
2. as a source of mutational processes in the germ cells, which is the basis for pathological processes of antenatal and postnatal development in the subsequent generations;
3. as a factor disturbing energy processes in the cells of vitally-important organs, which leads to:
   a) In relatively small amounts (20-30 Bq/kg), to disruption of regulatory processes in the organism, contributing emergence of the pathological processes and diseases, based on the latent genetic predisposition, due to the mutagenic effects including that of Cs-137, referring to the gametes in parental generations (dysregulatory effect of Cs-137), for example – congenital developmental defects, and the cardiac arrhythmia in children.
   b) in large amounts (more than 50 Bq/kg), to development of the necrobiotic changes in the cells with evidence of incorporated radionuclides, with destruction of their energy apparatus. For this example, the dilated cardiomyopathy.

In our opinion, the primary cause of increasing frequency of many diseases in the population, living in the territories damaged by the disaster of Chernobyl atomic station lies in this.

References

1. 15 лет после Чернобыльской катастрофы: последствия в Республике Беларусь и их преодоление. Национальный доклад / Под ред. В.Е.Шевчука, В.Л, Гурачевского. - Минск: Комитет по проблемам последствий катастрофы на Чернобыльской АЭС, 2001. - 118 с.

2. Амвросьев А.П., Баницкая Н.В. Ближайшие и отдаленные эффекты комбинированного воздействия иода-131 и цезия-137 в малой дозе на яичники животных // Доклады Академии наук Беларуси. -1992. - Т. 36. - № 9-10. - С. 855-857.

3. Бандажевский Ю.И. Патофизиология инкорпорированного радиоактивного излучения. - Гомель, Гомельский государственный медицинский институт, 1997. - 104 с.

4. Бандажевский Ю.И. Иммунная регуляция онтогенеза / Гомельский гос. медицинский ин-т. - Гомель, 1994. - 59 с.

5. Бандажевский Ю.И. Медико-биологические эффекты инкорпорированного в организм радиоцезия. Мн.: "Белрад", 2000. - 70 с.

6. Бандажевский Ю.И. Патология инкорпорированного радиоактивного излучения. - Мн.: БГТУ, 1999. - 136 с.

7. Бандажевский Ю.И. Радиоцезий и сердце (патофизиологические аспекты). - Мн.: "Белрад", 2001. - 62 с.

8. Бандажевский Ю.И., Переплетчиков А.М., Мишин А.В. Морфологическая и радиометрическая характеристика плодов, абортированных по медико-генетическим показаниям / Морфофункциональные аспекты действия радионуклидов на процессы антенатального и постнатального развития. Сборник научных трудов. - Гомель: ГОГМИ, 1998. - С. 28-31.

9. Бодяжина В.И., Кирющенков А.П., Побединский М.Н., Побединский Н.М. Влияние ионизирующей радиации на половые железы, беременность и внутриутробный плод. Медгиз. М. - 1962. - 182 с.

10. Бочков Н.П. Аналитический обзор цитогенетических исследований

после Чернобыльской аварии // Вестник Российской академии медицинских наук. - 1993. - №6. - С. 51-55.

11. Бочков Н.П., Аклеев А.В., Балева Л.С. Генетические последствия Челябинских и Чернобыльских радиоактивнкх загрязнений // Вестник Российской академии медицинских наук. - 1996 . - №6. - С. 64-72.

12. Варга С. В., Синицын П.В., Тарасенко Л.В. и др., Функциональная активность гипоталамо-гипофизарно-гонадной системы у самцов крыс в отдаленные сроки после рентгеновского облучения // Радиобиология. - 1993. - Т. 33. - № 3. - С. 337-341.

13. Ветух В.А., Малаховский Н.Н. Сравнительная оценка генетических эффектов равномерного внутреннего 137Cs и локального рентгеновского облучения крыс // Радиобиология. - 199I. - Т. 31. - Вып. 3. - С. 302-310.

14. Влияние радиоактивных веществ на половую функцию и потомство/Под ред. Д.И.Закутинского, М., гос. изд-во Медицинской литературы, 1963. - 242 с.

15. Гладкова А.И., Сидорова И.В., Карпенко Н.А. Системный анализ в оценке последствий облучения для репродуктивной функции // Актуал. пробл. влияния ионизирующ. излуч. на репроруктивн. функцию: Тез. докл. конф. Содружества Независимых Государств / РАМН Мед. радиол, науч. центр. - Обнинск, 1992. - С. 12 - 15.

16. Гончарова Р.И., Рябоконь Н.И. Частота аберраций хромосом и аномалий сперматозоидов у лабораторных мышей, содержащихся в загрязненных радионуклидами районах // Доклады Академии наук Беларуси. - 1994. - Т. 38. - № 4. - С. 84-87.

17. Гончарова Р.И., Рябоконь Н.И. Частота различных типов цитогенетических повреждений в половых клетках лабораторных мышей, содержащихся на радиационно-загрязненных территориях // Доклады Академии наук Беларуси. - 1995. - Т. 39. - №6. - С. 75-80.

18. Дыбан А.П., Баранов В.С., Акимова И.М. Основные методические подходы к тестированию тератогенной активности химических веществ // Арх. анат., 1970. - Т. 59.- № 10. - С. 89-100.

19. Золотухина Т.В., Кузнецов М.И., Костюк З.В. и др. Пренатальная диагностика как путь профилактики врожденных и

наследственных заболеваний // Вестник Российской Академии медицинских наук. - 1992. - №4. - С.14-20.

20. Индык Б.М., Парновская Н.В., Серкиз Я.И., Драган Ю.И. Сообщение 6. Физиологическое развитие и цитогенетические показатели у потомства крыс // Радиобиология. - 1991. - Т.31. - Вып. 5. - С.663-667.

21. Кириллова И.А., Новикова И.В., Арыдов Н.И., Налибоцкий Б.В. Частота пороков развития у зародышей человека в различный регионах Белоруссии // Здравоохранение Белоруссии. - 1990. - №6. - С. 53-55.

22. Лазюк Г.И,, Иванов В.И., Толарова М., Цейзель Э. Генетика врожденных пороков развития / В кн.- Перспективы медицинской генетики. Под ред. И.П. Бочкова. - М.: Медицина, 1982. - С. 187-240.

23. Лазюк Г.И., Николаев Д.Л., Ильина Е.Г. Мониторинг вроженных пороков развития у новорожденных южных районов Гомельской и Могилевской областей // Здравоохранение Белоруссии. - 1990. - №6. - С. 55-57.

24. Мамина В.П., Шейко Л.Д. Влияние малых и сублетальных доз ионизирующего излучения на состояние сперматогенного эпителия и выход доминантных летальных мутаций у мышей разных линий // Радиобиология. - 1993. - Т. 33. - №3. - С. 408 - 414.

25. Милютин А.А., Кирпичева Т.М., Лобанок Л.М. Влияние инкорпорированного цезия-137 на структурное состояние мембран эритроцитов // Радиобиология. - 1993. - Т. 33. - Вып. 2. - С. 302-305.

26. Романова Л.Д., Покровская М.С., Младковская Т.Б. и др. Особенности пренатального морфогенеза легких человека в зоне действия радиационных факторов после аварии на ЧАЭС // Онтогенез. – 1997. – Т. 28. - №1. - С. 41-48.

27. Столина М. Р., Соломко АЛ. Анализ репродуктивной функции самок лабораторных мышей CC57W/MY из чернобыльской и киевской популяций. // Актуал. пробл. влияния ионизирующ. излуч. на репродуктив. функцию: Тез. докл. Конф. Содружества Независимых Государств/ РАМН Мед. радиол. науч. центр. - Обнинск, 1992. - С. 69-70.

28. Цырельников Н.И. Гистофизиология плаценты человека. - Новосибирск. Наука, 1980. - 184 с.

29. Яговдик И.Н. Менструальная функция в условиях инкорпорации радиоцезия //"Чернобыль. Экология и здоровье". Научно-практический ежеквартальный сборник. Гомель. - 1998. - № 2 (6). - С. 88-94.

30. Залуцкий И.В., Жаврид Э.А., Машевский А.А. и др. Заболеваемость злокачественными новообразованиями в Республике Беларусь и смертность от них в 1992-2001 гг. // Здравоохранение. – 2003. – № 7. – С. 26-30.

31. Лелевич В.В., Дорошенко Е.М. Влияние воздействия инкорпорированных радионуклидов на фонд нейромедиаторов в головном мозге крыс / В кн.: Клинико-экспериментальные аспекты влияния инкорпорированных радионуклидов на организм. Под ред. Ю.И.Бандажевского, В.В.Лелевича. – Гомель. 1995. С. 74-88.

32. Дуда В.И., Дуда И.В., Сушко В.Я., Кулага О.К. Особенности полового созревания девочек, проживающих на территориях с повышенными уровнями радиации/ Достижения медицинской науки Беларуси. Выпуск 3. - 1998.

33. Мацюк Я.Р.,Гудинович С.Я.,Слободская Н.С., Михальчук Е.Ч. и др. Нарушения инкорпорируемыми радионуклидами становления у потомства структурно-метаболических и репродуктивных свойств женской половой системы и их профилактика /Достижения медицинской науки Беларуси. Выпуск 3. - 1998.

34. Бандажевский Ю.И.. Антонова Ю.В. Состояние репродуктивной системы женского организма в условиях воздействия радионуклидов // Бандажевский Ю.И., Лелевич В.В.,Стрелко В.В. и др. Клинико-экспериментальные аспекты влияния инкорпорированных радионуклидов на организм (под редакцией Бандажевского Ю.И.. Лелевича В.В.). - Гомель, 1995 .- Гл. 2. - С.24-34.

35. Политыко А.Д.,Егорова Т.М. Возможности цитогенетической базы данных в оценке тенденций и динамики поврежденный хромосомного аппарата у детского населения загрязненных радионуклидами зон Беларуси/ Достижения медицинской науки Беларуси. Выпуск 6. - 2001.

36. Лазюк Г.И., Румянцева Н.В., Политыко А.Д., Егорова Т.М. Анализ унаследованных и De NOVO структурных перестроек хромосом как один из методов оценки воздействия радионуклидов на наследственные структуры человека/Достижения медицинской

науки Беларуси. Выпуск 6. - 2001.

37. Наумчик И.В., Румянцева Н.В., Лазюк Г.И.Динамика частоты некоторых врожденных пороков развития в Беларуси / Достижения медицинской науки в Беларуси. Выпуск 6. - 2001.

38. Мацюк Я.Р., Абакумов В.З., Троян Э.И. и др. Особенности становления структуры и функции семенников у потомства при воздействии инкорпрорированных радионуклидов /Достижения медицинской науки Беларуси, Выпуск 2. - 1997.

39. Бандажевский Ю.И., Введенский Д.В., Лакудас Е.Л. Система мать-плацента-плод в условиях инкорпорации радионуклидов/ В книге Структурно-функциональные эффекты инкорпорированных в организм радионуклидов. Под редакцией проф. Ю.И.Бандажевского - Гомель, 1997. - С.119-141.

40. Марей А.Н., Бархударов Р.М., Новикова Н.Я. Глобальные выпадения Cs-137 и человек. Москва, Атомиздат, 1974. - 168с.

41. Здравоохранение в Республике Беларусь: Официальный статистический сборник - Минск: Белорусский центр научной медицинской информации Министерства здравоохранения Республики Беларусь, 2000. - 386с.

42. Официальный статистический сборник Министерства здравоохранения РБ за 2004 год.

43. Чернобыльская катастрофа: Причины и последствия (Экспертное заключение). В 4-х частях. Часть 3. Последствия катастрофы на Чернобыльской АЭС для Республики Беларусь / Под редакцией В.Б.Нестеренко / Международное сообщество восстановления среды обитания и безопасного проживания человека "СЭНМУРВ" Объединенный экспертный комитет (Минск-Москва-Киев). - Минск:"Скарына", 1992. - 207с.

44. Статистика Министерства здравоохранения Республики Беларусь. Демографические данные, данные по заболеваемости и смертности, показатели развития системы здравоохранения по регионам Беларуси с 1990 г., представленные в виде таблиц, диаграмм и карт / MED.by здравоохранение и медицинаская наука Беларуси.

45. Бандажевская Г.С. Состояние сердечной деятельности у детей, проживающих в районах, загрязненных радионуклидами / Медицинские аспекты радиоактивного воздействия на население,

проживающее на загрязненной территории после аварии на Чернобыльской АЭС: Материалы международного научного симпозиума. - Гомель, 1994. - С.27.

46. Бандажевская Г.С.Функциональные изменения миокарда в постнатальном онтогенезе при воздействии инкорпорированных радионуклидов. Автореферат диссертации. Москва, 1996. - 28с.

47. Бандажевский Ю.И.,Бандажевская Г.С. Влияние радиоактивных элементов,попавших в окружающую среду в результате аварии на ЧАЭС на состояние микоарда / В кн.:Клинико-экспериментальные аспекты влияния инкорпорированных радионуклидов на организм; Под редакцией Ю.И.Бандажевского, В.В.Лелевича. - Гомель, 1995. - С. 48-73.

48. Бандажевский Ю.И., Угольник Т.С., Вуевская И.В. Показатели антенатального и постнатального развития белых крыс при поступлении радионуклидов с пищей в период беременности // Здравоохранение Беларуси. - 1993. - №9. - С. 11-14.

49. Bandazhevsky Yu.I. Cs-137 incorporation in children's organs // Swiss. Med. Weekly, 133 ;p. 488-490, 2003.

50. Здравоохранение в Республике Беларусь/Официальный статистический сборник.- Минск, 2006.-275с.

51. Здравоохранение и медицинская наука Беларуси (Электрон, ресурс). Статистика Министерства здравоохранения Республики Беларусь.-1 декабря 2008г.- Режим доступа:http://stat.med/ by

52. Смертность в Республике Беларусь за 2004- 2005 гг. Официальный статистический сборник.- Минск, 2005./Составители: Министерство здравоохранения Республики Беларусь, сектор методологии и анализа медицинской статистики.- Минск : ГУ РНМБ,2006.-181с.

53. Состояние здоровья населения и организация медицинской помощи в Республике Беларусь. Статистика Министерства здравоохранения Республики Беларусь.-1 декабря 46 2009г.- Режим доступа:http://stat.med/by.

54. Доклад на коллегии министерства здравоохранения Беларуси. В. Жарко " Об итогах работы органов и учреждений здравоохранения на 2010 год".

55. Доклад зам. министра здравоохранения. Р. Чеснойть "Анализ состояния здоровья белорусских детей в 2009 году".

56. Бандажевский Ю.И., Зарянкина А.И. Содержание радионуклидов в организме детей первого года жизни в зависимости от вида вскармливания// Морфофункциональные аспекты действия радионуклидов на процессы антенатального и постнатального развития: Сборник научных трудов ГоГМИ. - Гомель, 1998. - С. 13-14.

57. Бандажевский Ю.И, Формирование костной системы зародышей белых крыс и золотистых хомяков в условиях экспериментального В1-гиповитаминоза // Архив анатомии. -1984.- № 11. - С. 88-92.

Section 2

Status of Reproductive Health of the Population, Living in the Territories of Ukraine, Damaged by the Consequences of the Accident at the Chernobyl Atomic Power Plant.

Chapter 2.1. § The main trends of birthrate in radioactively contaminated districts.

After the accident at the Chernobyl atomic power plant (CNPP) – the largest technological catastrophe in the human history, reproduction of population becomes an object of close attention for many researchers, in relation to growing unfavorable trends in some of its components [1-2]. It is especially urgent to study the factors, leading to reduction in the birthrate of population, living in the radioactively contaminated territories (RCT).

A huge amount of artificial radionuclides, fallen in the environment from the destroyed reactor, caused different radiological situations in the affected territories of Ukraine. In the first year after the accident at CNPP, the territories in which contamination of soil with Cs-137 exceeded 555 kBq/m², were classified as the districts of strict radiation control (SRC), and anti-radiation measures for the protection of population were introduced into them. In 1987, Poleski and Ivankov districts in Kiev oblast, Luginsky and Narodichi districts in Zhytomyr oblast, Kozeletsky, Repkin and Chernigov districts in Chernihiv oblast were classified as the areas of SRC. In 1988, the last three district of this list were excluded, and Ovruch district in Zhytomyr oblast was added. In the subsequent years, the composition of oblasts expanded to12, and of districts to 74. However, the levels of radioactive contamination of the first five districts remained most affected. All specified conceptions about the residence of Ukrainian population in RCT zone were identified in them [3], namely: the disposition, unconditional (obligatory) resettlement, guaranteed voluntary resettlement, and reinforced radio-ecological control. A significant number of people were envisaged to relocate from these districts in 1990-1992.

In the acute period after disaster, especially children suffered from irradiation to the thyroid gland by iodine radionuclide [4]. In all districts of SRC, the average dose levels exceeded the emergency criterion (30 cGy). And, they exceeded them also in adults in Narodichi and Poleski districts (52.6 cGy and 44.1 cGy, respectively). The cumulative doses of overall irradiation which, according to calculations, were received, on average data for each inhabitant in the districts for 1986-2000, amounted to 6.0-29.9 mSv.

In the first four years after the accident, inhabitants of the 175 residential settlements of districts in SRC received doses of total irradiation, exceeding the annual dose limit - 1 mSv/year, established in the conception of residence of the population in territories of Ukrainian SSR with elevated levels of radioactive contamination as a result of Chernobyl catastrophe (1991).

Demographics situations in the investigated districts until 1986 were characterized by high birthrate, fecundity, low migration, low mortality, urbanization and population density. Demographic indicators differed within insignificant fluctuations of the levels, which were comparable to the statewide values.

As a result of the Chernobyl catastrophe, the processes of reproduction of the population and the settlement changed drastically. The evacuation in 1986, and resettlement of inhabitants started in 1990, led to reduction in their number and deformation of the gender and age structure [5, 6]. For the first two months, after the accident at the Chernobyl nuclear power plant, 91.6 thousand inhabitants of two cities and 69 villages were evacuated from radioactively contaminated districts. The second wave of organized migration from RCT began in 1990 under the decisions of government. According to the official data of MES of Ukraine during 1986-1995, 112 residential settlements were resettled and about 163 thousand of people emigrated independently. In the following five years (1996-2000), relocation significantly decreased, and after 2000, it was reduced to isolated cases.

At the beginning of 2011, in the unconditional (obligatory) resettlement zone (zone II), 532 families remain to reside in Zhytomyr oblast (113 families of them, with children aged below 14 years in their composition), and in the disposition zone, where residence is prohibited, now there are one hundred and fifty "self settlers" [7]. At present, the main part of population in the areas of RCT live in the zones of guaranteed voluntary resettlement (zone III) and of reinforced radio-ecological control (zone IV).

Because of the resettlement and independent departure, proportion of women of reproductive ages was decreased in the population of districts of RCT. In 2000, their proportion was one third of the pre-accident level. The number of women in the age-related group of 20-29 years was reduced by 1.6 fold (reduced to about 63%), by whom 2/3 of all births of children were provided, whereas, in control, dynamics of this indicator had a positive tend (Figure 2.1.1.). The average age of the population increased by 2.5 years, which indicated intensification of depopulation processes.

Analysis of the natural dynamics of population showed that, for 1986-2000 years, in Ukraine birthrate was significantly reduced in comparison to the pre-accident period. This negatively influenced on the magnitude of crude birth rate (Table 2.1.1.).

The initial level of birthrate (1981-1985) in the districts of RCT corresponded to 14.1‰. For the first five years after the accident, it decreased from 13.7‰ (1986) to 8.8‰ (2000), which was 63% of the initial value. The most pronounced reduction in the birthrate (by 30%) was registered in the second year after the accident (Figure 2.1.2.). The reason for the sharp drop in the level of indicator was mass birth limitation of the population, particularly of the urban inhabitants, as a result of stress reaction to the Chernobyl event.

The lowest value of the birthrate was registered in 2000, in comparison to 1981-1985. The highest level of rate indicators decreased from 1991, in the uncontaminated territories as well as in the radioactively contaminated territories. The existing uniformity of dynamics of birthrate was formed against the background of amplification of destructive processes in the socio-economic life of society in 1990-1991, and their further amplification in the subsequent years (Figure 2.1.3.).

Dynamics of the crude birth rate depends on the features of structural changes in the population, particularly on the changes of proportion of women of reproductive ages (15-49) and the ratios of size of individual age groups within the range of this contingent. During 1986-2000, the age-specific birthrates in RCT decreased almost in all age groups, except for the youngest (15-19 years of age). In the second year after the accident, excessive birthrate was formed on account of senior women (45-49 years of age) and of the younger age group (15-19 years of age), but contributions of these age groups to the crude birth rate was small, and the indicated increase essentially does not influence the dynamics of indicator. During the investigated period in the radioactively contaminated districts (RCD), as well as in the uncontaminated districts since 1991, reduction in the birthrate was due to the more than 80%

Figure 2.1.1. Dynamics of the number of women in the ages of 20-29 years in radioactively contaminated and control districts of Ukraine for 1981-2000 years (the average indicator for 1981-1985 is taken as 100%).

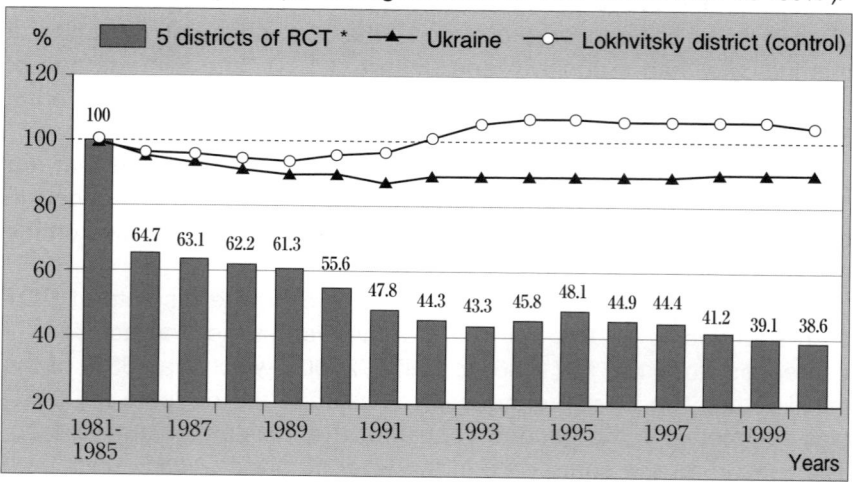

Note. * Ivankov, Poleski, Luginsky, Narodichi and Ovruch districts are included in the composition of districts.

Table 2.1.1. Dynamics of the crude birth rate in RCT and in control during 1981-2000 years.

territories	Crude birth rate, ‰			% changes in crude birth rate in comparison to 1981-1985	
	1981-1985	1986-1990	1991-2000	1986-1990	1991-2000
Luginsky district	15.0	13.8	12.7	−8.0	−15.0
Narodichi district	11.7	11.0	14.4	−6.0	+23.0
Ovruch district	13.8	12.2	10.7	−12.0	−23.0
Ivankov district	12.5	10.8	9.1	−14.0	−27.0
Poleski district	15.9	13.5	12.1	−15.0	−24.0
5 districts in RCT	14.1	12.9	10.9	−9.0	−23.0
Lokhvitsky district (control)	12.2	11.9	9.0	−3.0	−26.0
Ukraine	15.2	14.2	9.6	−7.0	−37.0

Source: Author's calculations based on the data of the State Statistics Committee of Ukraine.

Figure 2.1.2. Dynamics of the indicators of crude birth rate in the radioactively contaminated Ivankov district and uncontaminated Lokhvitsky district for 1981-1994 years (figures of 1981 taken as 100%).

The accident at the Chernobyl nuclear power plant

— ■ — Lokhvitsky district — ○ — Ivankov district

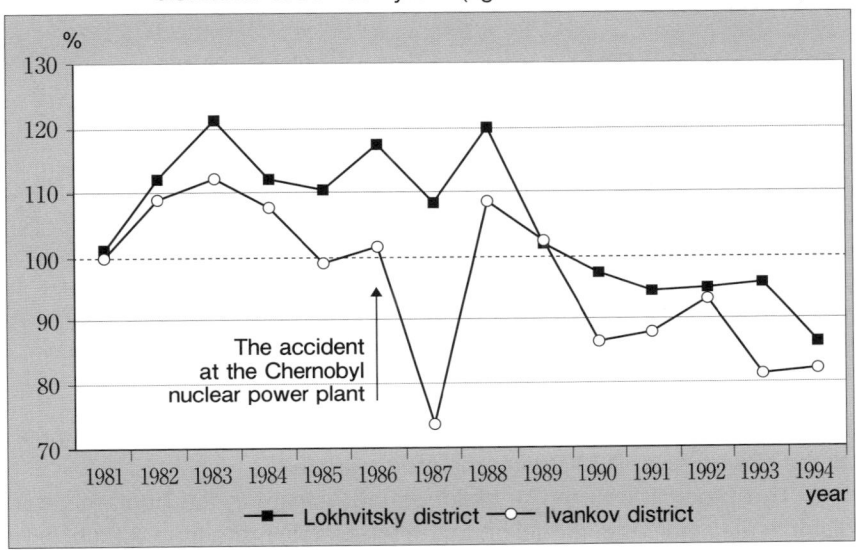

Figure 2.1.3. Dynamics of the crude birth rate of population and the stages of socio-economic transformations in Ukraine, during 1986-2007.

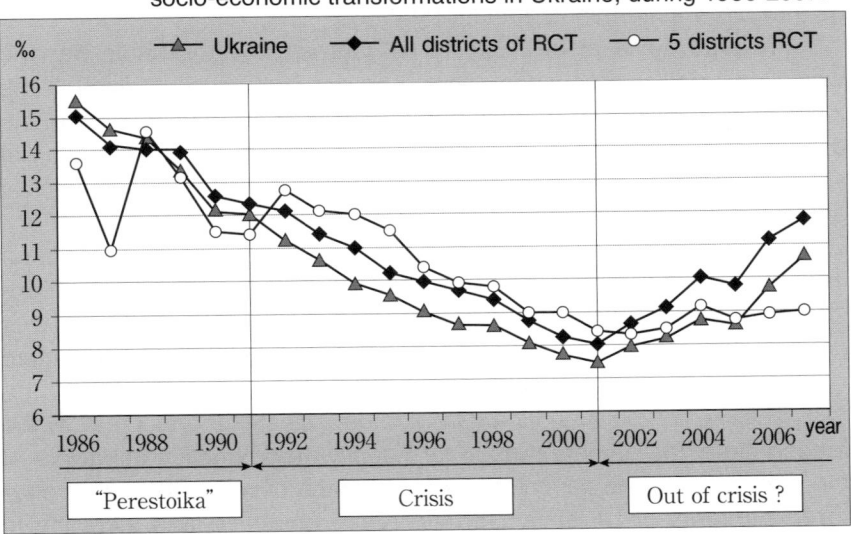

— ▲ — Ukraine   — ◆ — All districts of RCT   — ○ — 5 districts RCT

"Perestoika" | Crisis | Out of crisis ?

Figure 2.1.4. Contribution of individual demographic factors to the reduction in birthrate in radioactively contaminated districts (in percentages to the level of 1981-1985) for 1986-2000.

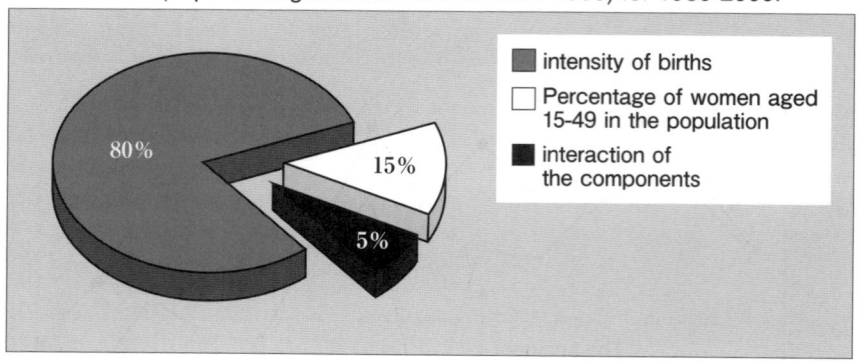

- intensity of births: 80%
- Percentage of women aged 15-49 in the population: 15%
- interaction of the components: 5%

decrease in the childbearing activity of women aged 20-34 years. Among all the newborns in RCT, firstborns predominated.

The precipitous drop of childbearing activity in the contaminated districts also indicates reduction in the total fertility rate from 2.2 children in 1986 to 1.2 children in 2001, including those in the urban settlements - from 1.8 to 1.1; in the rural area – from 2.3 to 1.4. During 1991-2002, most of the children (81-84%) were born to women under 30 years of age, i.e., childbearing activity of many women in RCT, and in the country as a whole, was terminated relatively early.

In 2000, level of birthrate in RCT crossed a threshold beyond which destructive processes occur, and consequence of which is the loss of prerequisites for the demographic and social development of the districts. This situation is considered by scientists as manifestation of social adaptation of the population, to altered conditions (ecologically and socio-economically) formed in the Post-Chernobyl period.

Using component analysis, it is determined that the contribution of intensity of births to the reduction in birthrate level in RCD during 1986-2000 was 80%, while, due to the structural factor, the birthrate was decreased by 15%, and the share of combined influence of both factors was 5% (Figure 2.1.4).

The opinion poll conducted in Ukraine indicates the fact that, at the present time, the primary reason for negative reproductive behaviors of the population is the severe financial situation of many families. Forty-three percents of Ukrainian female respondents named increase in

Table 2.1.2. The main indicators of birthrate of the population in Ukraine and radioactively contaminated districts in 1986-2007.

Years	Number of births per 1000 people			Average number of births per one woman		
	Ukraine	RCD*	RCD, in % to Ukraine	Ukraine	RCD	RCD, in % to Ukraine
1986-1990	14.1	13.4	95.0	2.2	2.1	95.5
1991-1995	10.8	11.1	102.8	1.6	1.7	106.2
1996-2000	8.4	9.0	107.2	1.2	1.4	108.3
2001	7.7	8.2	106.5	1.1	1.3	118.2
2002	8.1	8.7	107.4	1.1	1.3	118.2
2003	8.5	9.2	108.2	1.2	1.4	116.7
2004	9.0	9.8	108.9	1.2	1.4	116.7
2005	9.0	9.6	106.7	1.2	1.4	116.7
2006	9.8	10.5	107.2	1.3	1.5	115.4
2007	10.2	11.0	107.9	1.3	1.5	115.4

Note. * all districts relating to the damage by the accident at Chernobyl nuclear power plant in Ukraine.
Source: Author's calculations based on the data of the State Statistics Committee of Ukraine.

the level of income as the condition necessary for the births of desired number of children [8]. Housing conditions (17.9%), and absence of time of families for the upbringing of children (10.6%) play significant roles in the decisions of married couples, whether to have or not to have the desired number of children.

According to sociological monitoring conducted by the Institute Sociology, National Academy of Sciences of Ukraine [9], one tenth of the respondents living in zone II, and one sixth of zone III indicated the experienced aftermath of Chernobyl tragedy as a reason for not planning to have children in the future, whereas people in "clean" districts generally did not take this motive into account. In addition, more often than others, respondents in the population of RCT indicated economical factor in refusal of childbirth.

After a long period of steady reduction in the birthrate in affected districts, from 2002, its level began to increase gradually (Table 2.1.2.).

During 2002-2007, the crude birth rate was increased by 34.1% (in urban settlements - by 34.7%, and in villages - by 33.5%). For the last six years, childbearing activity of women in RCD increased in all age groups, especially in women aged 25-39 years with annual increases by

10%. These are the ages, when they give birth to the second or the third children.

Most of all, birthrate was increased in the urban women aged 30-39 years, which was associated with compensatory process of implementation of previously deferred births. There is evidence that a significant part of women had lost time for the births of first and second children to the corresponding age groups, and in this connection, in 2002-2007, some "shift" of births of the first children from the age-related group of 20-24 years old to the age group of 25-29 years old, of the second children – from the age-related group of 25-29 years old to the group aged 30-34 years, and of the third children – from the group aged 30-34 years to the group aged 35-39 years occurred.

Compensatory implementation of previously deferred births was caused by two oppositely directed processes: on one hand – some improvement in the welfare of population, and on the other hand – gradual social adaptation to new conditions of life, and in addition, implementation of measures by directions of pronatalist on demographic policies (in effect from April 1, 2005 ponderable one-time assistance at child birth).

The specific stimulating factor improving birthrate was temporary replenishment with childbearing contingent, on account of the entry into reproductive age of people born in 1983-1986. Analysis of age-related childbearing activity according to the type of settlements of population in RCD revealed some peculiarities of the mode of birthrate of urban and rural women.

Among rural women, a distinctly pronounced rise in the childbearing activity in the age group under 24 years was observed. In the rural terrain of RCD, reproductive activity of women under 20 years of age was twice as high as, and that of the age group of 20-24 years was 1.5 times higher than, those in the urban settlements.

That is to say, majority of women in the rural terrain of RCT (60%) implement their fertility function under 25 years of age. Urban women led in the total births of children of second and third queues between the ages of 30-39 years. And, it rather means, that urban women more often postpone giving birth to the first child, and the countryside traditionally has a propensity for early births and early marriage. Urban women who had low starting indicators, since 2002, were actively included in the childbearing process in the subsequent years, especially of 35-44 years of age.

Changes in the levels of birthrate, which occurred in RCD in the last decade, came with a significant transformation of age-related model of mass reproductive behavior. Young people today start processes of childbirth later than those two decades ago. Not only young women but also socially more mature women – older than 25 years, provide a significant part of the current level of birthrate.

Trend of changes in the age-related model of birthrate in RCD can be traced in dynamics of the indicator of the average age of maternal contingent, which practically did not changed for the first 12 post-accident years: 24.1 years old in 1986 to 23.8 years old in 1998. A rapid and steady increase in this indicator in RCT occurred in 1998-2007. During this period, it rose by 1.7 years and in 2007, was 25.5 years old.

In Ukraine, starting from 2005, demographic policy of oblasts for the material supports to the families with young children was intensified.

One time assistance at childbirth was dramatically increased to one of the highest amount in Europe, which was raised again in 2008. However, the public opinion poll in order to clarify their attitudes toward the government conducted activities showed that the weighty one time assistance at childbirth did not in any way influence the childbearing attitude in most respondents (87.4%) [10]. As confirmed by the experiences of many countries in the world, which tried to quickly solve the problem of low birthrate, one time emergency measures does not yield sustainable effects. Moreover, specialists predict that in the next decade, reduction in the proportion of women in the most active age of childbearing is anticipated, which bring Ukraine new problems, since the impact of structural factor will be very large.

In this way, the mode of birthrate of inhabitants in radioactively contaminated districts of Ukraine, which was formed in the post-accident period, has a threatening nature for the reproduction of popu-lation. According to the international scale of basic demographic indicators, the current level of birthrate is assessed as extremely low, although some "higher" values are preserved against the nationwide background. Emerging in 2002, positive trends in birthrate were caused by the increased childbearing activity of women aged 25-39 years, on account of compensatory implementation of previously deferred births. The main factors which favored increase in the birthrate in radioactively contaminated districts, and in Ukraine as a whole, were the temporary replenishment with childbearing contingent on account of the entry into reproductive ages of people born in 1983-1986, and measures of demographic policy conducted from 2005.

Chapter 2.2. § Characterization of reproductive losses of the population and their contribution to the dynamics of birthrate.

The main limiting factor for the reduction in birthrate of inhabitants in RCT in the post-emergency period was the number of children born. In conditions of low birthrate, reproductive losses[1] (RL) affect efficiency of reproduction of the population.

> 1 : The index takes into account, cases of spontaneous abortion, artificial abortion for medical indications, the number of stillbirths and the number of dead children aged 0-6 days per 100 desired pregnancies.

After the accident at Chernobyl nuclear power plant, steady increase in RL-index was observed in the radioactively contaminated districts. The contribution of RL to reduction in the crude birth rate was no more than 3.5% in 1987, and in 1994, ranged within the limits of 9.4-25.0 %, depending on the districts. Thus, the heaviest negative impact of the index on birthrate was identified in Narodichi (25.0%), Poleski (18.6%) and Ivankov (15.5%) districts. In the radioactively "clean" territories, the level of birth rate was reduced by reproductive losses by 1.1% on average.

Quantitative features of RL in the individual districts show that substantial excess of RL (excess above the control were 5.3 and 8.1 times, respectively) was formed in Luginsky and Poleski districts even in 1986-1990 (Table 2.2.1.). Since 1991, negative trend of increasing indices was observed in all the investigated districts, except for Narodichi district of Zhytomyr oblast [11].

In the structure of RL, more than 85% of the cases were spontaneous abortion. The frequency of this pathology in the general population of Ukraine, according to various authors, ranges from 5 to 25%. [12, 13]. However, in most cases, early abortions, which account for about 8% of all pregnancies, remain unrecognized [14]. According to the official statistical materials, the average rate of registered cases of early abortion in the investigated districts for 1986-1999, was in the range from 3.7 to 5.6% of all pregnancies, and formally did not exceed the upper limit registered in the world [15].

Table 2.2.1. Quantitative characterization of reproductive losses in the radioactively contaminated and conditionally "clean" districts in the pre- and post-accident periods, per 100 desired pregnancies (%).

Districts	Reproductive losses			Figures of the ratio to 1983-1985		Excess of reproductive losses in comparison to 1983-1985	
	1983-1985	1986-1990	1991-1999	1986-1990	1991-1999	1986-1990	1991-1999
Luginsky	3.54	5.93	5.99	1.68	1.69	+2.39	+2.45
Narodichi	6.29	4.98	4.76	0.79	0.76	-1.31	-1.53
Ovruch	1.67	2.54	5.52	1.52	3.31	+0.87	+3.85
Ivankov	4.32	5.33	9.73	1.23	2.25	+1.01	+5.41
Poleski	3.87	7.50	8.26	1.94	2.13	+3.63	+4.39
5 districts RCT	2.68	4.21	6.94	1.57	2.59	+1.53	+4.26
Lokhvitsky	4.10	4.55	7.76	1.11	1.89	+0.45	+3.66

In 2000, as compared with 1983-1985, the rate of RL in the investigated districts increased 2.4 times, while in the uncontaminated territories – increased only 1.5 times. The increase in the rate of RCD was statistically significant ($p<0.05$). Average annual rate of increase in the analyzed districts, was 0.27 cases of RL per 100 desired pregnancies on average. The highest value of the index was recorded in 1991-1992 (exceeding the pre-accident level more than 2.5 times)[16].

Since 1986, statistically significant ($p<0.05$) increase in the level of relative risks of RL was registered in the investigated territories, on account of spontaneous abortions and the death of children in the early neonatal period, which correlated with total collective effective dose of irradiation to the population [17].

It is established that women who live in radioactively contaminated residential settlements and accumulated a certain dose of total body irradiation, have an increased risk of occurrence of spontaneous abortion to them as compared with those who live in radioactively uncontaminated territories [18].

Increase in the level of RL occurred against the background of deteriorating health of pregnant women. Since 1987, in RCD, persistent trend toward increasing frequency of late gestational toxicosis (1.5-2.3 times) and gestational anemia (10.0-13.8 times) was observed. The consequence of this was the increase in the incidence of complications of delivery. Incidence of unfavorable outcomes of pregnancy in women was increased almost 2.1 times due to spontaneous abortions. Since 1986, spontaneous abortions in the 22-27 weeks of gestation are more frequently registered. In 1989-1990, among all spontaneous abortions, their share was 19%, while in the radioactively clean districts - 10% [11]. One of the main causes of spontaneous abortion, and therefore of RL, are the congenital developmental defects.

In 2000, UNSCEAR of UNO concluded that the increase in the number of congenital anomalies, developmental defects and RP, which was shown in some researches of the scientists in Ukraine and Belarus, could not be attributed to the radiological influence as a result Chernobyl catastrophe. This conclusion was made on the basis of knowledge of the world radio-biology about dose-dependent effect of ionizing radiation.

However, it should be noted that the official doses of irradiation to Ukrainian population were significantly underestimated, because of the methodological inconsistency and errors in the dose estimation in 1986 [19]. In the Ukrainian methods, they were calculated not by the methods of systematic analysis of radiation accidents as it is done all over the world, and a low value of dose coefficient (9.4 $\mu Sv/Bq \cdot m^2$) was simply assigned to the emergency dose of 1986 for the whole Ukraine without any scientific justification. This was done in order to belittle the aftermath of the accident at Chernobyl atomic station. The irradiation dose of Ukrainian population in the year of accident (1986) was evaluated only as a few percent of the lifetime received dose, whereas in the Russian Federation it was evaluated as 90%. At the most modest estimates, people really received or will receive for their lives at least 10 rem of radiation beyond the established norm of 7 rem. According to the risk theory, this means that one person out of 1000 people who received this dose, or their descendants will suffer [19].

Assessing the revealed changes, one can state that the long residence of people in radioactively contaminated territories is a risk factor to increase the level of reproductive losses and therefore, to reduce the birthrate. However, for the correct evaluation of influence of the existing radiation factor on the development of embryo, information about individual doses of irradiation to population is necessary. To our regret, in Ukraine, at the present time this information is absent.

At the same time, the index of reproductive losses are influenced by other factors except for the radiation factor, in particular, deterioration in the reproductive health of future parents, age of the mother, incomplete registration of the cases of reproductive losses and others.

The obtained results indicate that the processes of birthrate of the inhabitants in the radioactively contaminated territories has a direct relationship to the consequences of the Chernobyl catastrophe, and their tendencies acquired threatening character for the reproduction of population. The levels of indicators of birthrate, the total fertility rate and reproductive losses, suggest that adaptation of investigated human population to the unfavorable conditions of the ambient environment is reduced. Improvement of the situation with regard to the birth rate requires the decisions at government level.

The most feasible ways to increase the birthrate in radioactively contaminated territories are:
1. Implementation of the necessary measures for anti-radiation protection to the population;
2. Conducting activities contributing to protection of health of mother and child;
3. Preserving each desired pregnancy, provided the physiological course of pregnancy and normal development of the fetus;
4. Implementation of measures directed to reinforcement of reproductive health of the population.

References

1. Демографічна криза в Україні. Проблеми дослідження, витоки, складові, напрями протидії / За ред.. В. Стешенко. – К.: Інститут економіки НАН України, 2001. – 325 с.

2. Медико-демографическая специфика радиационно загрязненных регионов Украины / Г.Л. Глуханова, И.А. Курило, Е.П. Рудницкий, Л.В. Задоенко // Экологическая антропология. Ежегодник. – Минск: Белорусский комитет «Дети Чернобыля», 2001. – С. 50-54.

3. Про правовий режим території, що зазнала радіоактивного забруднення внаслідок Чорнобильської катастрофи. Закон України від 27 лютого 1991 р. № 791а-XII / За ред. Дурдинця В., Самойленка Ю., Яценка В., Яворівського В. // Соціальний, медичний та протирадіаційний захист постраждалих в Україні внаслідок Чорнобильської катастрофи: Зб. законод. актів та нормативних документів. 1991-2000 роки. 2-ге вид. - К.: Чорнобильінтерінформ, 2001. - С. 297-308.

4. 4. 20 лет Чернобыльской катастрофы. Взгляд в будущее: Национальный доклад Украины. – К.: Атика, 2006. – 224 с. 59

5. Доценко А.И. Региональное расселение: проблемы и перспективы. – К.: Наукова думка, 1994. – 214 с.

6. Гунько Н.В., Дубова Н.Ф., Омельянець М.І. Міграція жителів України у зв'язку з Чорнобильською катастрофою: історичний аспект // Екологія довкілля та безпека життєдіяльності. - 2004. - № 6. - С. 19-23.

7. Информационно-справочные материалы по вопросам преодоления последствий Чернобыльской катастрофы / Информационно-аналитические материалы Кабинета Министров Украины на парламентские слушания. – К.: 2009. – 59 с.

8. Здоровье детей и женщин в Украине. – К.: Кабинет Министров Украины при поддержке ЮНИСЕФ, ПРООН и др. межд. Организаций, 1997. – 127 с.

9. Лавриненко Н. Адаптация института семьи к постчернобыльской

ситуации // Чернобыль и социум (Выпуск шестой). – К.: Центр социальных экспертиз и прогнозов Института социологии НАНУ, 2000. – С. 81-99.

10. Семья и семейные отношения в Украине: современное состояние и тенденции развития. – К.: ТОВ «Основа-Принт», 2009. – 248 с.

11. Дубовая Н.Ф. Влияние последствий Чернобыльской катастрофы на рождаемость населения радиоактивно загрязненных территорий Украины и пути ее улучшения: Автореф. дис… канд. мед. наук: 14.02.01 / Институт гигиены и медицинской экологии им. А.М. Марзеева АМН Украины. – К., 2002. – 19 с.

12. Стешенко В. Состояние репродуктивного здоровья в Украине (медико-демографический обзор). – К.: МЗ Украины, Институт экономики НАН Украины, 2001. – 68 с.

13. Гойда Н.Г., Дудина О.О., Моисеенко Р.О. Охрана здоровья детей и женщин. – К.: Здоровье, 2001. - С. 221-242.

14. Репродуктивные потери (клинические и медико-социальные аспекты) / В.Н. Серов, Г.М. Бурдули, О.Г. Фролова, З.З. Токова, Т.Н. Пугачева, В.В. Гудимова. – М.: Триада-Х, 1997. – 188 с.

15. Состояние пострадавшего населения Украины и ресурсы охраны здоровья через 15 лет после Чернобыльской катастрофы: Статистическо-аналитический справочник. Часть II. – К.: НДВП «ТЕХМЕДЕКОЛ», 2001. – С. 185.

16. Дубовая Н.Ф. Оценка риска репродуктивных потерь у населения территорий Украины, загрязненных радиоактивными выбросами // Довкілля та здоров'я. – 2001. - № 3. С. 42-46.

17. Дубовая Н.Ф. Современные тенденции формирования уровня младенческих потерь на радиоактивно загрязненных территориях Украины // Экологическая антропология. Ежегодник: научное издание мат. XI межд. научно-практ. конф. "Экология человека в постчернобыльский период" 3-5 ноября 2003 г., Минск. - Минск: Белорусский комитет "Дети Чернобыля", 2004. – С. 109-112.

18. Тимченко О.И., Линчак О.В. Ионизирующая радиация в малых дозах и здоровье населения (анализ литературы и результатов собственных исследований). – 2006. - № 1. – С. 39-46.

19. Пик «постчернобыльской» заболеваемости // Газета 2000. – 2008. - 10 января. – С. 16-17.

Conclusion

Certainly, all aspects of problems of human reproduction in the territories damaged by the radiation impact in consequence of Chernobyl catastrophe cannot be covered in a small book. It is evident that existence of demographic catastrophe due to the high mortality and low birthrate of the population should be recognized. The low birthrate is also, to a great extent, due to the mortality of the human organisms in the early stages of their development. One can state a variety of processes, contributing to the occurrence this situation. One of its main causes was ignoring the danger of actually existing radiation factor for the human organism, as a result, effective measures for anti-radiation protection of population, first of all, at the State level, were not implemented adequately.

Based on the results of scientific research, it can be concluded that continuous presence of radioactive element Cs-137 in the ambient environment and therefore, in the human organism causes energy deficit in the cells of vitally important organs, which leads to development of severe pathological processes, resulting in fatal outcome.

In particular, the indicated radiation factor is one of the causes of male and female infertility, acting on all parts of the reproductive system, including the central nervous system and endocrine organs.

Decay of radioactive agents causes mutation in the germ cells of parents, which finds its negative manifestation in the subsequent generations, in some cases incompatible with life.

The mother-fetus system is also very sensitive to radioactive exposure. Radionuclide Cs-137 infiltrated into this system contributes to the intrauterine death of embryo and emergence of congenital developmental defects. It should be noted that registration of the pathological processes in human embryo in early stages of intrauterine development is quite difficult. For this, organization of medical, genetic and pathomorphological investigations, with participation of specialists competent in the matters of pathology of intrauterine development is required. Essential component for this kind of investigations is determination of the content of radioactive agents in the fetal organism and organs, and also in the placenta.

Realization of the disorders of embryogenesis, induced by the radiation exposure, is possible not only in the period of intrauterine development but also at the stage of postnatal development of organism. It is important to understand to maintain the principle in setting etiopathogenic diagnoses of the diseases recorded in children, adolescents, and adults.

To our deep regret, processes of intrauterine development of the human organism in conditions of the impact of incorporated radionuclides, are yet poorly investigated, which does not allow to fully develop and implement the effective measures for the prevention of pathology in the antenatal and postnatal ontogeny, including in the adult organism.

It should also be noted that in the real situation, there are combined impacts of a number of factors of external environment on the developing organism. Nicotine and alcohol, as well as narcotic agents should be included in this kind of factors, providing negative impacts on the processes of reproduction. Unfortunately, they are fairly widely distributed among the population in the districts contaminated with radionuclides, and undoubtedly, intensify the recent pathogenic effects on the human organism. To some extent, the disregarded radiation impact hides behind these factors as the main cause of high morbidity and mortality, including those in the intrauterine period.

In this regard, it should be emphasized that in addition to radiation protection measures, with all the possible means, alcohol consumption of the population living in the territories contaminated with radioactive elements should be reduced, and reduction in the number of smoking individuals should also be facilitated.

Medical problems directly associated with the tremendous socio-economic problems, occurred in the territory of former USSR, due to its collapse. Chernobyl has created socio-economic crisis, which in turn, exacerbated the Chernobyl situation.

Nowadays, it is difficult to have optimistic views in respect of the prospects for existence and development of the human population, directly facing radiation impact. Medical duty obliges us to continue to fight for the lives of people, using all our capabilities. We have no right to step aside, leaving them alone with deadly threats.

LIST OF ABBREVATIONS

Rem - off-system unit of measurement of equivalent dose of irradiation

kBq/m² - a unit measuring the density of contamination by radioactive nuclides of soil by the International System of Units

mSv - a unit of measurement (by SI units) of equivalent dose

UNSCEAR - United Nations Scientific Committee on the Effects of Atomic Radiation

UNO - The United Nations Organization

Regions of SRC - regions of strict radiation control

RCD - radioactively contaminated districts

RCT - radioactively contaminated territories

cGy - a unit of measurement (by SI units) of the absorbed dose of ionizing radiation

ChNPP - The Chernobyl atomic power plant

MES of Ukraine - The Ministry of the Emergency Situations of Ukraine

NASU - National Academy of Sciences of Ukraine

RL - reproductive losses

NCRPU - The National Commission for Radiation Protection of Ukraine

Cs-137 - Cesium-137

Ba-137 - Barium-137

Xe-137 - Xenon-137

I-131 - Iodine-131

Ig M - Immunoglobulin M

Ig G - Immunoglobulin G

INDEX

Pages

Preface of the authors 69

Section 1 Incorporated radionuclide Cs-137 and the processes of human reproduction. 71

Chapter 1.1. Radiological and demographic situation in the Republic of Belarus before and after the Chernobyl disaster. 71

Chapter 1.2. Female reproductive system in condition of incorporation of radio-cesium. 76

Chapter 1.3. Male reproductive system under the condition of incorporated radio-cesium. 80

Chapter 1.4. Mutagenic effects of radio-cesium. 82

Chapter 1.5. Features of incorporation of radio-cesium in the periods of pregnancy and lactation. 83

Chapter 1.6. Pathology of the antenatal and postnatal development with incorporation of radio-cesium. 86

    1.6.1. Assessment of congenital defects in the human being with account of incorporation of Cs-137. 86

    1.6.2. Assessment of embryo-fetogenesis in laboratory animals at incorporation of radio-cesium in the period of pregnancy. 92

Chapter 1.7. Placenta and incorporation of radio-cesium. 100

Chapter 1.8. Mutual endocrine relations in the mother-fetus system with incorporation of radio-cesium. 102

Chapter 1.9. Radiation-toxicity syndrome of fetus and newborn. 104

Section 2 Status of Reproductive Health of the Population, Living in the Territories of Ukraine, Damaged by the Consequences of the Accident at the Chernobyl Atomic Power Plant. 121

Chapter 2.1. The main trends of birthrate in radioactively contaminated districts. 121

Chapter 2.2. Characterization of reproductive losses of the population and their contribution to the dynamics of birthrate. 130

Conclusion 136

［著者］
ユーリ・I・バンダジェフスキー（Yu. I. Bandazhevsky）
1957 年、ベラルーシ、グロドノ州生まれ。
1980 年、国立グロドノ医科大学卒業。1982 年、病理解剖の臨床研修を終え、ジュニア研究者として中央科学研究所に入所、同研究所所長に就任。1990 年、ゴメリ医科大学を設立し、1999 年まで学長、病理学部長を務める。ベラルーシコムソモール賞、アルバート・シュバイツァーのゴールドメダル、ポーランド医学アカデミーのゴールドスターを授与される。本研究の成果が、「放射線は人体の健康にほとんど影響しない」というベラルーシ政府の方針に反したことから、入学試験の賄賂汚職の容疑で逮捕され、8 年間の禁固刑に処せられる。支援者の陳情によって、5 年に軽減されたが、出獄後もベラルーシでは復職できず、フランス、リトアニアを経て、現在はウクライナ（キエフ）に在住。エコロジー健康調整分析センター理事長。
2009 年、欧州放射線リスク委員会（ECRR）レスボス会議からエドワード・ラッドフォード記念章受賞。

N・F・ドウボバヤ（N. F. Dubovaya）
ウクライナ保健省シュピーク記念学士教育国立医学アカデミー準教授（食物衛生学および子どもと未成年者衛生学講座）。
医学修士、上級科学研究員。

［訳者］
久保田 護（くぼた・まもる）
チェルノブイリの子供を救おう会代表。
茨城大学名誉教授（工学博士）。
大正 13 年（1924）9 月生れ、昭和 18 年（1943）9 月旧制水戸高等学校卒業、東京帝国大学入学、昭和 21 年（1946）9 月同学第二工学部卒業、国産鉄工株式会社、下妻第二高等学校、日立工業高等学校、茨城大学工学部に勤め、平成 4 年（1992）4 月茨城大学名誉教授、平成 15 年（2003）4 月叙勲、勲三等瑞宝章。

放射性セシウムが生殖系に与える医学的社会学的影響
チェルノブイリ原発事故　その人口「損失」の現実

2013 年 4 月 1 日　第 1 刷発行

著　者　ユーリ・I・バンダジェフスキー／N・F・ドウボバヤ
訳　者　久保田 護
発行者　上野良治
発行所　合同出版株式会社
　　　　東京都千代田区神田神保町 1-28
　　　　郵便番号　101-0051
　　　　電話　03（3294）3506 ／ FAX　03（3294）3509
　　　　URL　http://www.godo-shuppan.co.jp/
　　　　振替　00180-9-65422
印刷・製本　新灯印刷株式会社

■刊行図書リストを無料進呈いたします。
■落丁乱丁の際はお取り換えいたします。

本書を無断で複写・転訳載することは、法律で認められている場合を除き、著作権および出版社の権利の侵害になりますので、その場合にはあらかじめ小社あてに許諾を求めてください。

ISBN 978-4-7726-1089-6　NDC464　210 × 148
© Mamoru Kubota, 2013